American Folk Medicine

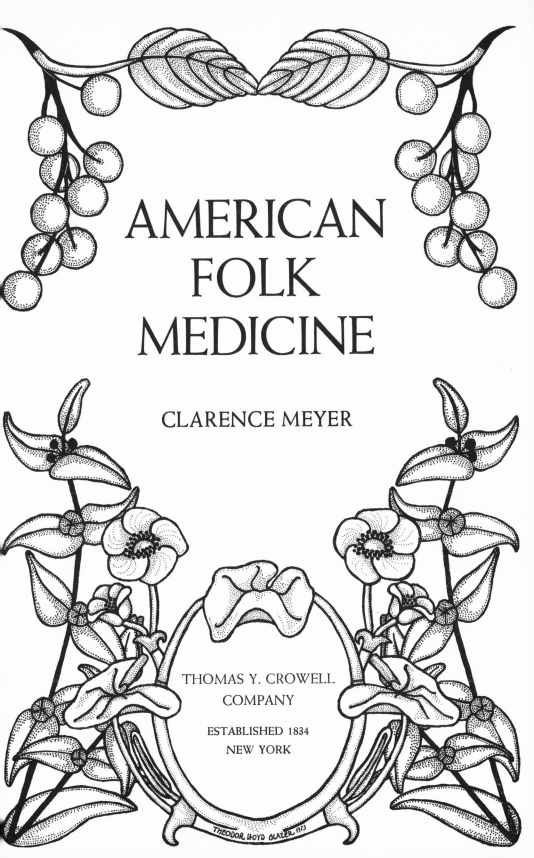

AMERICAN
FOLK
MEDICINE

CLARENCE MEYER

THOMAS Y. CROWELL
COMPANY

ESTABLISHED 1834
NEW YORK

THEODOR LLOYD GLAZER 1973

DESIGNED BY ABIGAIL MOSELEY

MANUFACTURED IN THE UNITED STATES OF AMERICA

ISBN 0–690–06693–7

1 2 3 4 5 6 7 8 9 10

Library of Congress Cataloging in Publication Data

Meyer, Clarence, comp.
    American folk medicine.

    Bibliography: p.
    1. Folk medicine—United States. I. Title. [DNLM: 1. Folk-
lore. 2. Folklore—History. WZ 309 M612a 1973]
R152.M49   615'.882'0973   73-4300
ISBN 0-690-06693-7

In Memory of
My Mother and Father

Special Notice

This book is intended solely as a record of folk medicine and does not represent an endorsement of any recipe, nor does the author or publisher vouch for any claims made for them.

Contents

AUTHOR'S NOTE   xi

EARLY AMERICAN PRACTITIONERS   1

COMMON CONDITIONS TREATED
IN AMERICAN FOLK PRACTICE   23

BIBLIOGRAPHY   279

COMMON AND LATIN NAMES OF PLANTS   283

Author's Note

Folk medicines are still relied upon in remote areas of America. While medical conditions have been greatly improved in 250 years, there still is only one doctor for every 600 persons, according to a 1971 American Medical Association report.

Simple kitchen products, garden vegetables and well-known botanicals such as caraway and fennel seeds, chamomile flowers, sage, rosemary, dandelions, spices, etc., merit greater use as home medicine than some of the easy-to-take (and overtaken) potent drugs that are being so freely dispensed without prescriptions in almost any type of store. The wider use of harmless home remedies for distresses beneath the doctor's attention would alleviate some of the unnecessary burdens of overworked doctors.

Until the advent of heart transplants, artificial kidneys, antibiotics, etc., physicians of the ages advised their students not to shun folk medicines when they proved to be of value. This advice began with the ancient civilizations. Herodotus relates in his works how the Babylonians had a custom of placing their sick persons in a structure in the public marketplace where all could see them. Everyone was obliged to ask the patient how he felt and what he had done to help himself—and to make suggestions to aid his recovery. When a treatment was recommended that had cured someone before, the patient was taken home immediately and treated by the same method. In this manner, the knowledge of herb remedies was spread throughout the kingdom.

Hippocrates, the father of medicine, said, "One should not

abhor asking the simple folks whether a thing is a good remedy, as many drugs have been found often enough by plain people and by mere chance, rather than by planned scientific investigation." Paracelsus, often referred to as the father of chemistry, said that he acquired many of his most effective remedies from various sources, including monks, barbers, surgeons, midwives, hangmen, gipsies and herb-collecting old women. Centuries later, Dr. Benjamin Rush advised his students, "When you go abroad to practice, always take with you a memorandum book, and whenever you hear an old woman say such and such herbs are good, or such a compound makes a good medicine, or ointment, put it down, for, gentlemen, you may need it."

In more recent years a Virginia doctor of allergies told an assembly of family doctors how often the most puzzling allergy patients responded with exceptional results from injections of nonspecific extracts made of common plants. He said there was no scientifically proven reason why the treatment worked. He believed when a physician's best efforts failed, it was justifiable to use nonofficial remedies if they helped. It is said that the operation of acupuncture, the Chinese anesthesia, is still unexplainable after some 2,000 years of use in folk practice. During a recent trip to China, Western doctors were amazed at its success.

A noted professor of pharmacy said that if modern science had been more open-minded about the ageless secrets of medical folklore, antibiotics would have been brought to light many years earlier. He also pleaded for the collection and cataloguing of all herbal-medical folklore because it is rapidly disappearing. He believed the most ridiculous sounding recipes merited scrutiny.

Many recipes appearing in *American Folk Medicine* were gathered over a period of more than two generations, and their sources are often unknown as they were intended originally only for family use. There are countless slight variations in recipes for common conditions such as hiccups, coughs and colds, wounds, bruises and sprains, aches and pains, etc. This book is limited to the recipes most commonly used. Recipes with doubtful ingredients are not listed. About the mid 1800s, many recipes became predominately of chemical composition. The author believes such materia medica was derived from professional practice rather than domestic sources. Recipes in *American Folk Medicine* are limited mainly to ingredients found in the old-time household or available at the general store and from itinerant peddlers. Recipes containing foreign ingredients originated in Europe, while those containing native plants are usually of Indian origin.

The recipes in this book are presented as they were originally written, although minor changes in diction and puntuation have been made for the sake of clarity.

The author wishes to emphasize that extravagant medical claims were often made by rustics, pioneer settlers, frontiersmen and undereducated practitioners to instill faith in their concoctions. Throughout the ages faith has been considered a helpful ingredient in medical practice. It still is a helpful factor in conditions requiring the full cooperation of the patient. Placebos would be quite useless if the doctor prescribing them did not have the faith or confidence of his patient. It must also be realized that "sure cure" recipes oftentimes afforded only temporary relief or palliated a condition diagnosed by untrained home doctors. If it were true that a recipe was a sure cure, infallible cure, sovereign cure, etc., there would have been no reason to list a multitude of other recipes for the same distress.

Time is often an important factor in medication, and a physician should be consulted for all conditions requiring his services.

American Folk Medicine

Early American Practitioners

In 1721, Boston, which was then nearly 100 years old, had only one European-graduated doctor practicing in the city. Few foreign doctors ventured to leave civilization for a new land of uncertainties where familiar drug supplies were scarce or unavailable. For some 200 years after the first colonists arrived, there were no hospitals or medical schools. Old World recipes printed in almanacs and newsprints were the main sources of medical information available to the general public. A few imported drugs could sometimes be purchased in shops that sold farm tools, seeds, guns, dry goods, dyestuffs and groceries. Oatmeal was sold by the ounce. It was used as a poultice and sometimes taken internally. Chinese tea, when available, was also considered a medicinal. The tea leaves were boiled the usual way and the strained-off liquid discarded. The soggy tea leaves were eaten with a bit of salt and butter.

Indian medicines were essential to the early colonists, especially during the long winter months when few ships came from the Old World. Squaws sold native botanicals in the streets of the settlements and were often asked to help the ailing. Indian healers gained local repute for their successes in treating the sick. Joe Pye was an Indian healer who traveled through the colonies curing typhus fever by promoting copious perspiration with a brew made of the roots of a common weed that is still known as Joe Pye weed, or *Eupatorium purpureum.*

The New World developed an assortment of practitioners. People with the slightest knowledge practiced medicine either as a side line or as full-fledged doctors, depending upon capability and demands for their services. A young man wishing to enter the profession apprenticed himself to someone who had already established a practice sufficiently to use the title Physician. The apprentice was generally required to do a variety of jobs as a sort of tuition fee. He pulverized botanicals and chemicals, helped make pills, tinctures, sirups, prepare salves, liniments, etc. He swept floors, ran errands, followed the doctor on sick calls, and sometimes he was left with the patients to carry out the doctor's instructions. When business was slow, a doctor served as veterinarian or made up alcoholic bitters, elixirs, special formulae for man or beast, aphrodisiacs or longer-life concoctions. His products were dispensed by himself or sold to itinerant peddlers. Much of the learning of the apprentice depended upon his observation and memory. Diplomas were not issued—the apprentice "graduated" when he felt he knew all the tricks of the trade.

Prominent people also practiced medicine. Their medical education was generally acquired from foreign medical literature or contact with foreign-trained physicians. William Salmon's huge volume, *Botanology: or, the English Herbal* (1710), took the place of a college course as a means of learning medicine and pharmacy. A smaller volume, *Medicina Britannica* (1746), by Thomas Short, M.D., was also a popular source of medical knowledge in colonial times. Dealers occasionally announced the arrival of shipments of books and they were eagerly sought by those who could read and afford them.

Governor Edward Winslow and Governor John Winthrop had their own private practices and their special list of prescriptions for the ailing. Winthrop's son, John, Jr., Governor of Connecticut, was considered an outstanding physician in the colonies. He made house calls, prescribed by letter and had his own cure-all. Alice Morse Earle wrote in *Customs and Fashions in Old New England* (1893), "All the early parsons seem to have turned eagerly to medicine, the Wigglesworths [parsons] were famous doctors. President Hoar of Harvard College, President Rogers, President Chauncey, all practiced medicine. The latter's six sons were all ministers and all good doctors too." Educated practitioners of New England perpetuated Old World practices. Opium, mercury, arsenic, antimony, vitriols, etc. were used freely and bloodletting was resorted to in almost any condition.

In desperate times medical help often had to be sought wherever it could be found. Some slaves proved to have a remarkable aptitude in the healing arts. A slave named Caesar won fame for remedies curing poisons. The following news item appeared in the *Carolina Gazette* in the 1700s: "The General Assembly had purchased the negro Caesar's freedom and granted him a pension of one hundred pounds per annum during life, as a reward for the discovery of the means by which he acquired so much celebrity in curing persons who had swallowed poison or been bitten by a rattlesnake." Various species of native gentians were known in colonial times as Sampson snakeroot because a slave named Sampson cured snake bites with the roots of these plants.

Earle wrote: "A good old Connecticut doctor had a negro servant, Primus, who rode with him to help him in his surgery and shop. When the master died, Doctor Primus started to practice medicine himself and proved extraordinarily successful throughout the country."

Slaves doctored themselves. Like the Indians they had always lived close to nature and quickly learned the properties of plants. Peter Smith, an Indian doctor, noted, "This root, Abela or Trumpet Weed [unidentified], the Africans give to make the wenches amorous and more fruitful. It is supposed to excite venereal desires."

In 1749, the General Assembly of South Carolina in Charleston passed an act prohibiting slaves being employed by physicians or apothecaries to concoct poisons or administer medicines of any kind, under threat of death.

In 1793, a plague of yellow fever in Philadelphia spread beyond the control of regular doctors. In desperation, Dr. Rush devised a system he believed to be a "grand specific" to control the epidemic. Because of the shortage and differences in opinion of some doctors, Dr. Rush employed apothecaries, private citizens, women and "even colored people" to go about and prescribe his method. Dr. Rush wrote, "The success of his 2 negroes in curing the disease was unparalleled by what was called regular practice."

Women also became practitioners. As they dabbled in herbal concoctions for the care of their families, it was natural that those with special abilities were sought to help the ailing in their communities. Margaret Jones was a very successful doctor in Charlestown, Massachusetts, but was one of the first victims of a relic of the Dark Ages brought from the Old World. Margaret was hanged in 1648. The fact that she could bring about wonderful cures with simple roots and herbs was sufficient evidence she possessed the diabolical powers invested in witches!

While doctoring women did not fare well in Puritan settlements,

3

their help was most invaluable to pioneers living near them in the wilderness. The following occurred about 1777 in New Hampshire and was recorded by Samuel Thomson: "There was an old lady by the name of Benton lived near us, who used to attend our family when there was any sickness. At that time there was no such thing as a doctor known among us; there not being any within 10 miles. The whole of her practice was with roots and herbs, applied to the patient, or given in hot drinks to produce sweating, which always answered the purpose. When one thing did not produce the desired effect, she would try something else, until they were relieved." After a severe winter and many hardships living in a barn, while a log cabin home was being constructed, Thomson's mother became seriously ill; "she was carried to Mrs. Benton's for her to take care of, where she remained for several weeks, during which time, by using means as this old lady prescribed, she recovered."

Aunt Prudie was another unsung heroine of the wilderness country. She lived in Mississippi in the 1800s and was already a very capable midwife when still very young. There were no "diploma doctors" within fifty miles of the place where Aunt Prudie lived, so the backwoods folk relied on her for medical assistance as well as for childbirth delivery. Aunt Prudie braved many nights alone on horseback to reach the bedside of an expectant mother or an ailing child. Her reputation and successes eventually spread over a wide area of the South. Old-timers said she delivered 2,914 babies in 65 years of practice and nursed back to health many thousands of the sick. Aunt Prudie's medicines consisted mainly of medicinal plants gathered from nearby fields, although much of her medical knowledge was acquired from "book doctors."

Midwives were an ever-at-hand source of medical help in colonial settlements as well as in the backwoods. The profession of the midwife is the oldest in man's history. It began in remote antiquity when females had to help each other in times of difficult childbirth. Only in recent times have male physicians delved into obstetrics, and many of their basic methods were obtained from the midwife. Tombstone records of midwives reveal deeds of the past. Inscriptions on a stone in an old burial ground in Charleston, South Carolina, claims Elizabeth Phillips delivered some 3,000 babies. A Mrs. Lydia Robinson of New London, Connecticut, delivered 1,200 babies in a 35-year period without losing a single mother or baby.

One of the most singular personalities in American folk medicine was self-educated Samuel Thomson. His M.D. title was bestowed on him by patients for his remarkable successes in curing where "fashionable" doctors failed with bloodletting, blistering, mercury, antimony, vitriols, and other popular European medicaments and methods of that day.

Samuel Thomson was born in Alstead, New Hampshire, in 1769. He spent most of his early life of poverty and hardship in wilderness country. His father, a very stern religious man, took Samuel to drive cows to pasture and tend geese when he was not yet 4 years old. The boy amused himself tasting, smelling and chewing various plants found in fields and nearby woods. One weed caused the boy to vomit. He induced other boys to eat the weed—it acted upon them in the same way. In later years, while working in the fields, Samuel again found the weed and dared an adult to eat it. Shortly after, the man became violently ill, perspired, then vomited copiously. After about 2 hours the man ate a hearty meal and returned to work in the field. Samuel named this little plant emetic herb—it became the "No. 1" herb in his practice.

When Samuel was 10 years old, he had an opportunity to attend school for a month. He wrote, "The weather was cold and the going bad [the school was about a mile from home], which caused me to make very slow progress in my learning; but the chance we considered a great privilege for the country was new and people poor, and the opportunity for children to get learning very small."

Because of Samuel's interest in plants, at the age of 16 his parents wanted him apprenticed to a root doctor. This failed because Samuel did not have enough "learning." He confided, "I now gave up all hopes of going to any other business and tried to reconcile myself to spend my days in working on a farm, which made me very unhappy. I had little learning and was awkward and ignorant of the world, as my father had never given me any chance to go into company to learn how to behave, which caused me great uneasiness."

Samuel Thomson's medical "learning" began in 1788 when he was 19. The learning consisted of a serious accident, experiences with various fashionable doctors and root doctors, self-treatment, family illnesses, nursing, and his mother's death. Thomson married in 1790. In the following year he learned the horrors of a difficult childbirth, the miseries of its aftereffects and later the diseases of childhood.

Since Samuel Thomson's wife needed periodic medical care after the birth of their first baby, he decided to allow a young root doctor to live on his farm. Thomson learned much from the doctor in the 7-year period he lived there. He gradually assumed most of the care of his family while the doctor "got into the fashionable mode of treating his patients, by giving them apothecary's drugs, which made him more popular with the faculty."

Gathering herbs in season became one of the chores of the Thomson family "for I found by experience that an ounce of preventative was better than a pound of cure." Thomson continued gathering his own medicine after he became a practitioner. He often made long trips seeking supplies of botanicals.

In later years he advised that the following stock of medicinals always be kept at hand by the average family for one year: 1 ounce of emetic herb; 2 ounces of cayenne; 1 to 2 pounds powdered bayberry bark of root; 1 pound poplar bark; 1 pound ginger; 1 pint rheumatic drops. The word *rheumatic* apparently meant pains in general (both internal and external) as well as rheumatism. (Thomson's recipe for rheumatic drops is given in the section of this book entitled "Pain.")

After the fashionable root doctor left the Thomson farm, the family had little trouble until the birth of their third son. Thomson recorded: "At the birth of our third son, my wife was again given over by the midwife. Soon after the child was born, she was taken with ague fits and cramp in the stomach; she was in great pain and we were much alarmed at her situation. I proposed giving her some medicine, but the midwife was much opposed to it; she said she wished to have a doctor and the sooner the better. I immediately sent for one and tried to persuade her to give something which I thought would relieve my wife until the doctor could come; but she objected to it, saying that her case was a very difficult one and would not allow to be trifled with; she said she was sensible of the dangerous situation my wife was in, for not one out of twenty lived through it, and probably she would not be alive in 24 hours from that time. We were thus kept in suspense until the man returned and the doctor could not be found, and there was no other within 6 miles. I then came to the determination of hearing to no one's advice any longer, but to pursue my own plan. I told my wife that as the midwife said she could not live more than 24 hours, her life could not be cut short more than that time, therefore there would be no hazard in trying what I could do to relieve her. I gave her some warm medicine to raise the inward heat and then applied the steam which was very much opposed by the midwife; but I persisted in it according to the best of my judgment and relieved her in about 1 hour, after she had lain in that situation above 4 hours, without anything being done. The midwife expressed a great deal of as-

6

tonishment at the success I had met with, and said that I saved her life.

"These things began to be taken some notice of about this time and caused much conversation in the neighborhood. My assistance was called for by some of the neighbors and I attended several cases with good success." Word of Thomson's successes had spread beyond the family circle. He wrote, "I began to be sent for by people of this part of the country so much, that I found it impossible to attend to my farm and family as I ought; for the cases I had attended I had received very little or nothing, not enough to compensate me for my time; and I found it to be my duty to give up practice altogether or to make a business of it." After consulting his wife and friends, Thomson decided: "I am convinced that I possess a gift in healing the sick, because of the extraordinary success I have met with, and the protection and support Providence has afforded me against the attacks of all my enemies. Whether I should have been more useful had it been my lot to have had an education and learned the profession in the fashionable way, is impossible for me to say with certainty; probably I should have been deemed more honorable in the world; but honor obtained by learning, without a natural gift, can never in my opinion make a man very useful to his fellow creatures."

Epidemics frequently ravaged cities and villages of early America. In 1793, an epidemic of yellow fever returned to Philadelphia for the second time, killing some 4,000 people in a 3-month period. Dr. Thatcher wrote that it "baffled the skill of the oldest and most judicious physicians."

Dr. Thomson recorded in 1805 that "a very alarming disease prevailed in Alstead and Walpole, which was considered the yellow fever and was fatal to many who were attacked by it. I was called on and attended with great success, not losing one patient that I attended; at the same time those who had the regular physicians, nearly one half of them died." Although Dr. Rush prescribed bleeding twice a day for 10 days, Thomson thought, "It appeared to me very extraordinary to bleed 20 times to cure the most fatal disease ever known." Dr. Thomson did not hesitate to attend any case no matter how contagious it was. He recommended "keeping a piece of ginger root in the mouth and chew it like tobacco, swallowing the juice. This should be done by all who are exposed to any contagion, or are attending on the sick, as it will guard the stomach against taking the disease."

7

Dr. Thomson attended numerous cases and recorded an epidemic of 1808: "In the fall of this year the dysentery or camp distemper, as it was called, was very prevalent in Jericho and was so mortal that all but two who had the disease and were attended by the doctors died, having lost above twenty in a short time. The inhabitants were much alarmed and held a consultation to advise what to do; and being informed by the young man above mentioned, that I was at home, they sent an express for me and I immediately made arrangements to comply with their request. In 24 hours I started and arrived there on the third day after, and found them waiting with great anxiety for me, having refused to take anything from the doctors. I had an interview with the selected men of the town, who had taken upon themselves the care of the sick; they informed me that there were about 30 then sick and wished me to undertake the care of them. I agreed to take charge of them on condition that I could have two men to assist me; this was complied with and I commenced my practice upon 30 in the course of 3 days. The disorder was most distressing of any that I have ever witnessed. One man had been speechless for 6 hours and was supposed to be dying; but on my giving him some medicine to warm him, he seemed to revive like an insect that was warmed by the sun after having laid in a torpid state through the winter. I had but little medicine with me and had to use such as I could procure at this place. I found the cause of the disease to be coldness and canker [infection]; the digestive powers being lost, the stomach became clogged so that it would not hold the heat. I made use of red pepper steeped in a tea of sumach leaves, sweetened, and sometimes the bark and berries, to raise the heat and clear off the canker, which had the desired effect. After taking this tea, those who were strong enough, I placed over a steam, as long as they could bear it, and then put them to bed. Those who were too weak to stand, I contrived to have sit over a steam; and this repeated as occasion required. To restore the digestive powers, I made use of cherry stones, having procured a large quantity of them, that had been laid up and the worms had eaten off all the outside, leaving the stones clean. I pounded them fine, then made a tea of black birch bark, and after cleaning them by putting them into this tea and separating the meats from the stone part, made a syrup by putting from 2 to 3 oz. of sugar to 1 quart of the liquor; this was given freely and answered a good purpose. I continued to attend upon my patients, aided by those appointed to assist me, and in 8 days I had completely subdued the disease.

They all recovered except 2, who were dying when I saw them. I gave the same medicine to the nurses and those exposed to the disease, as to them that were sick, which prevented their having the disorder. The same thing will prevent disease that will cure it."

Dr. Thomson's mode of steaming was imitated by root doctors and some fashionable doctors, much to his chagrin. He stated, "Though they [doctors] condemned me and my practice, they were willing to introduce it and take the credit to themselves as an important discovery."

Dr. Thomson's successes became legend. His services were sought by individuals with long-standing illnesses and by patients given up by regular doctors. Thomson found it increasingly difficult to attend his ever-growing practice especially during epidemics. To alleviate this situation he devised a system of treatment so "that every family should practice for itself; that a knowledge of the medicine and its administration should be as familiar to every family as the knowledge and use of their daily bread." The system was sold to individuals or groups, giving them "rights" to use his discoveries. Small towns without doctors also purchased the "rights."

Dr. Thomson's "novel mode of practice" engulfed him in more and more conflict with a medical faculty that was now gaining power. Dr. Thomson wrote: "They [New York doctors] have succeeded in getting a law passed by their legislature to put a stop to quackery, as they call all practice, except by those who get a diploma from some medical society established by law; depriving all others the right of collecting their demands for medical practice; and they have also gone one step further than any other state by making it penal for anyone who is not of the regular order to sell medicine to the sick, imposing a fine of $25.00 on all who offend; thus taking away from those who are so unfortunate as to be sick, all the rights of determining for themselves who shall employ to cure them, or what medicine they shall make use of. The Medical Society of Pennsylvania made an attempt to get a similar law passed in that state; but the good sense of Governor Shultz put a stop to it, for which he is entitled to great praise. After they had managed to get it through the legislature, he refused to sign it and returned the bill with his reasons; the principal of which was that he considered it altogether unconstitutional; and it is to be hoped that the enlightened statesman and scholar, now Governor of New York, will use his influence to stop the interested and monopolizing schemes of the medical faculty in that important and enterprising state."

9

Much of Dr. Thomson's extraordinary successes may be accounted for from the early experiences he acquired in doctoring himself, his family, friends, neighbors and people in nearby towns. His lifelong interest in and experimenting with native medicinal plants gave him a unique advantage in the choice of plants to use with patients. His inherent talent as doctor-nurse, combined with an ability to follow therapeutic procedures according to patient reactions, also was a major factor in curing critical cases that were sometimes given up to die. Dr. Thomson's ingenious ability to improvise in emergencies was proved in the epidemic at Jericho, when his regular supply of medicine became exhausted.

For almost a century after *New Guide to Health: or, Botanic Family Physician* (1831), Thomsonian-type books under various titles have extolled, copied or imitated the doctor tutored by hardships and experiences.

BOOK DOCTORS

European medical books were an invaluable source of help to practitioners as well as households in colonial America. The most popular publications available to the general public were: Theobald's *Every Man His Own Physician* (1764), Culpeper's *English Physician* (1652), and Buchan's *Domestic Medicine* (1769). Theobald's small book dealt with a few common ailments. Culpeper's book, an astrological herbal, was more informative and eventually became the most reprinted herbal since printing was invented. Buchan wrote that his book was "an attempt to render medical art more generally useful by showing people what is in their own power both with respect to the prevention and cure of diseases, chiefly calculated to recommend a proper attention to regimen and simple medicine." *Domestic Medicine* was repeatedly reprinted until superseded by American publications in the 1800s.

Numerous English and German almanacs published treatments for a variety of ailments. Franklin's *Poor Richard's Almanack* printed a recipe for dissolving kidney stones with lemon juice; recipes for gout; cures for worms; remedies for dropsy and yellow jaundice; a "certain and speedy" remedy for pimples; health care of children; a cure for glanders in horses; etc.

After the American Revolution, printing expanded rapidly in New England, and presses were moved westward as fast as towns mushroomed into cities. Many publishing companies and small print shops joined the assorted medical practitioners to print advice and recipes for self-medication. Early so-called American medical books contained a scant mention of native medicinals, the books being more or less duplicates of oft-repeated European publications. Schoepf's *Materia Medica Americana* and Thatcher's *Pharmacopoeia* were among the earliest to reveal the virtues of native American plants. Rafinesque's volumes, *Medical Flora of the United States* (vol. I, 1828; vol. II, 1830), added new species and medicinals, clarified many doubtful common names, and listed native drug plants that could be substituted for expensive or hard-to-get foreign drugs. Rafinesque traveled thousands of miles by foot into fields, wilderness and mountains to get firsthand information for his prodigious researches, drawings and collections.

Medical Flora of the United States lists contemporary writers with the author's appraisals. The following is a partial list with Rafinesque's remarks:

Barton, *Vegetable Materia Medica of the United States.* "Another costly work mentioning about 1 plant in 40 of North America. Descriptions short and flimsy."

Coxe, *American Dispensatory,* 7th edition, 1827. "Useful compilation, few original indications on plants."

Cutler, *Plants of New England.* "Rude attempt, many botanical mistakes, some medical indications."

Elliott, *Sketch of the Botany of Carolina and Georgia,* 3 volumes, 1818 to 1822. "Under that modest title we have the best Flora of the Southern States, full of New Species, good descriptions and with several medical indications."

Henry, *Medical Herbal,* 1814. "Empirical, erroneous in names, descriptions, facts and figures, some medical facts, and local names."

Hunter, *Narrative,* 1824. "Another impostor, he has given a list of western medical plants with Osage names, not to be depended upon or ascertained."

Rafinesque incurred the wrath of certain members of the faculty with his criticisms and varied writings. A modern source states his works were effectively suppressed by Asa Gray.

An interesting record of folk medicine was made in the early 1800s by practitioners popularly known as Indian herb or root doctors. These self-proclaimed and often self-educated doctors printed limited editions of pamphlets or miniature books containing information gleaned from contemporary sources and lore gathered from frontier people and Indians. It will never be known how many of these publications were lost because of the precarious lives of their owners.

Peter Smith's *Indian Doctor's Dispensatory, Being Father Smith's Advice Respecting Diseases and Their Cure* (1812), is one of the earliest as well as the rarest publications of its kind. Smith, the pioneer farmer, preacher and doctor wrote, "My father, old Hezekiah Smith, of Jersey, was always, since I could remember him, a home old man, or Indian Doctor, with whom, in my raising, I contracted ideas, practice and experience that never left me." Smith believed that "Nature had made him a physician; and to the best of his recollection, he always remembered everything that he has ever met with in a medical way, that he has counted valuable." He called himself an Indian doctor "because I have incidentally obtained a knowledge of many of the simples used by the Indians; but chiefly because I have obtained my knowledge in the like manner that the Indians do. I have by continued observation come to be of opinion that our best medicines grow in the woods and gardens."

Books of the Indian doctors were sold mainly in new settlements and probably were prized for their size and ready-at-hand medicines. While school-trained doctors adhered to Old World doctrines and materia medica, Indian doctors advocated the use of native American plants. Dr. D. Rogers, author of *The American Physician* (1824), stated: "The means of health are scattered so profusely around us in almost every field and forest—placed as it were, within reach of every hand that will deign to accept. . . . Exotic vegetables may perhaps prove useful, especially if naturalized by cultivation in our own soil, in our own climate; but it is at least probable, if not certain, that our own native plants are abundantly sufficient to answer all the medical demands of our country."

The Indian herb doctor claimed intimate contact with Indian medicine men. John Monroe wrote in his most informative small book, *The American Botanist and Family Physician* (1824): "For the attainment of his object [his book] he travelled; to this end he has labored; and for years plied himself in the wilds of America among the natives of the forest where he has undergone all the horrors and deprivations incident to savage life in order to collect and bring together that knowledge which should be instrumental in saving the lives and preserving the health of his fellow creatures. Whilst among the Indians, the author was a particular intimate and confidant of a native Indian, who had been instructed in all the arts

12

of civilized life and had received the advantages of a liberal and polite education, being regularly bred a physician in the medical department of the Pennsylvania University established at Philadelphia; at once the most flourishing and respectable institution of the kind in the United States and hardly excelled by any in Europe."

Pierpont F. Bowker's tiny book, *The Indian Vegetable Family Instructer* (1836), stated, "Recipes have been carefully selected from Indian prescriptions and from those very persons who were cured by the same after every other remedy had failed."

Doctor L. Sperry, author of *The Botanic Physician* (1843), derived much of his medical information from nine different tribes of Indians. Dr. Sperry, like many other Indian doctors who were also preachers, stressed moderation in food, drink and rest, and concluded: "To preserve steadily in this course is often times more than half the cure. Above all, add to the rest—for it is not, I assure you, nor will it be labor lost—that old fashioned medicine, prayer, and have faith in God who killeth and who maketh alive, who turneth man to destruction, and who saith return, ye children of men."

The House Surgeon and Physician (1820), by Dr. William Hand, was perhaps the earliest American-approved book for self-medication. It was recommended by N. Smith, M.D., a professor of the theory and practice of physics, surgery and midwifery in the medical institution of Yale College, and by M. F. Gogwell, M.D., president of the Connecticut Medical Society (1818).

Dr. Hand wrote: "Physicians and Surgeons cannot be present in every place; nor can they alone do everything which should be done for those to whom they are called. The sick and wounded must depend much on nurses and attendants; and almost every individual thing which is done for the sick is influenced by the notions or prejudices of the attendants. How important, then, that the means of information relating to the healing art, be extended to every one who may suffer, or who can watch. There are cases also where medical aid cannot be obtained; and shall the sufferer lie without relief?"

Dr. Hand said of broken bones: "There is, in most country villages, some person who pretends to the art of setting bones. Though in general, such persons are very ignorant, yet some of them are very successful; which evidently proves that a small degree of learning, with a sufficient share of common sense and a mechanical head, will enable a man to be useful in this way."

Bloodletting was considered an essential part of most treatments by the profession. *The House Surgeon and Physician* gave detailed instructions for cupping, bloodletting and the use of leeches. The book named some native plants used in domestic practice, but the majority of the prescriptions were those used by so-called regular doctors.

Gunn's *Domestic Medicine: or, Poor Man's Friend* (1830) became the first American book version of the family-type doctor. Unlike most previous publications for home medication, Dr. John C. Gunn explained in simple language body functions and the effects of exercise, emotions and intemperance upon health. Gunn's book was a predecessor of a long line of family-style medical publications that appeared in the late 1800s and early 1900s. Gunn's *Domestic Medicine* became an indispensable part of many households in small settlements, outlying farms and log cabin homes of settlers in the Midwest where the books were printed. Lillian Kruerger wrote in *Motherhood on the Wisconsin Frontier* (1946): "The mother's ingenuity had to meet pioneer medicinal deficiencies, and she did well enough with her knowledge of wild plants, berries, barks, flowers and roots. These she collected throughout the seasons—gladly assisted by the grandmother —and dried and labeled them to be kept and used upon short notice. In some of the settlements Dr. Gunn's medical volume was almost as sacred as the Bible and a great blessing during those hard years."

In 1857 Dr. Gunn published a revised and much enlarged *New Domestic or Family Physician* which became the most popular medical publication of its time. By 1885 it reached its 213th edition. Many German printings were also made. Dr. Gunn's revised book included Latin names of medicinal plants which were lacking in the early editions. The new edition revealed a change in therapeutic practices, with far less bloodletting and an increase in the use of chemical drugs.

Families living in the new territories or wilderness sections of the Midwest had to be more or less self-sustaining according to the distances they lived from towns or cities where stores, trade shops and supplies were available. Dr. Gunn's medical book served well where doctors were unavailable, but the comforts of home and farm necessities depended much upon the capability of the pioneer settlers. Dr. Chase's *Recipes: or, Information for Everybody,* became an immediate success because his book included besides its medical advice, a variety of do-it-yourself instructions and recipes for every phase of home, farm or business. Chase was for a number of years in the grocery and drug business. He studied medicine and graduated as a physician when he was 38 years of age. Dr. Chase's first publication consisted of a pamphlet of a few pages printed in 1856. As he traveled, he collected recipes from all classes of professional business men, mechanics, furriers, farmers, etc. His later books were packed with an assortment of information for every type trade. His book included recipes for "minor medical conditions" and "rational treatment of pleurisy, inflammation of the lungs, and other inflammatory diseases, and for general female debility and irregularities," as they were described in the 1874 edition. Dr. Chase's book went through many editions, and copies are still found in old homesteads.

Medical advice was dispensed in cookbooks, domestic economy books, encyclopedias, farm books and government publications, as well as in newspapers, magazines and almanacs. In the early 1900s numerous ponderous volumes were printed on domestic medicine; advice included conduct in the sick room, development and control of passions, chastity and inchastity, love, courtship and marriage, etc.

HOME DOCTORS

Home remedies and self-medication often meant life or death to people living in sparsely settled communities or in isolated cabins far from assistance or medical help. Choking, broken bones, hemorrhages, poisoning, gangrene, snakebites, fevers, gunshot or arrow wounds had to be treated at once by the best known means. The kitchen, garden and woods were often the sole sources of materia medica for emergencies as well as lingering illnesses.

Since family life began, the care of babies in health and sickness was a natural instinct endowed to all mothers. This trait established her as the doctor and nurse of her household. A mother's qualifications consisted of inborn common sense and the skills her own mother taught her. Good medical, cooking and household recipes were treasured and preserved from one generation to another.

Being the cook for the family, mother knew energy and health depended much upon the operation of the stomach. Hearty meals supplied vigor for manual workers and lighter foods sustained the sedentary. Mother's cooking skill was best demonstrated in times of illnesses. She had a store of recipes for easy-to-digest liquid or semi-liquid foods to fit conditions of all ages. Wheys, barley water, toast or apple water, soups, gruels, panadas, porridges, calve's feet jelly, etc., were important articles in home medication. Easily assimilated medicines—infusions and decoctions—were also considered important as a means of conserving and strengthening the vital forces of the debilitated. There is a congruous relationship between food plants and nontoxic medicinal plants grown in the same soils. Food plants generally contain a considerable proportion of starches, while medicinal plants contain greater concentrations of therapeutic properties. Both type plants have a natural affinity to the human body that has thrived upon them for so many ages.

Mother did not have a name for vitamins or minerals, yet it had long been known what foods supplied energy to restore health. A favorite recipe for the convalescent was a cup of rich broth made by boiling a piece of beef until all the essence was extracted from it. Now it is generally conceded that such a broth does have power to restore strength. The beef broth abounds in the element potassium, which plays a vital role in muscular action. Patients weak from the loss of a large amount of potassium from diarrhea or vomiting are greatly benefited by the old-time meat concentrate treatment.

Mother believed that like her home the body needed periodic cleaning out. Skin pores needed sweating, especially when "obstructions" or colds threatened. The kidneys needed occasional flushing, and the bowels were also given timely and seasonal purging. Nature is exceptionally bountiful in medicinal and food plants to help keep man inwardly clean.

Mother had various spring tonics to use after a long winter spent semihibernating and living in stuffy and often smoke-filled rooms. There were cooling and "blood thinning" root beers and herb teas for summer; heady brews and ciders for fall and winter; and smacking bitters for the flagging appetites of the aged.

Mother knew nothing about viruses or germs—she could only see as far as her glasses allowed. She was more concerned about "purifying bad blood" and building bodily resistance rather than in fighting a little "bug" that could not be seen.

Mother's home doctoring often prevented a variety of disorders or at least abated their severity simply because she "did something" as soon as symptoms appeared. Sympathetic care and meticulous, devoted nursing methods also contributed much to home-doctoring successes. Many recipes were intended to ease or comfort the patient, allowing inherent healing powers to bring about a normal cure. Mother often gave *tisanes,* medicinal-flavored beverage, in order to keep her patient in bed for a recuperating rest. Miraculous cures have been known because of the infinite attention only a mother or a loved one can give.

FOLK MATERIA MEDICA

Self-medication with folk materia medica was very different than self-medication with potent modern drugs. The majority of articles used in folk medication were quite harmless and often effective therapeutics when discreetly used.

Infusions and decoctions were the important media of medication. In the early days when water was taken from rivers and questionable sources, it was boiled. A few sprigs of aromatic herbs were thrown in the boiling water to disguise bad flavors. Some infusions became popular native teas. Pleasant-tasting herb teas were often used when taking pulverized botanicals that could not be boiled because of their volatile nature or because the botanicals did not yield their virtues in boiling water. Pennyroyal tea was taken as a beverage during medication in the belief the drink would "cause the medicine to have a pleasant operation." Hard-pressed pioneers found that the stomach would bear more of a tea made with the delicately scented life everlasting (*Gnaphalium polycephalum*) than it would tolerate plain water. They discovered a variety of uses for a single native botanical. Dr. Hand wrote in 1820: "By different preparation and management, boneset herb (*Eupatorium perfoliatum*) may be made to produce a variety of effects. A strong tea prepared by long steeping, or by boiling, taken freely while warm, may, according to the quantity, be made either to produce perspiration and assist in raising phlegm from the lungs, or to purge, or to vomit; taken cold and in more moderate quantity, it gives strength. In one or other of these methods, it may be useful in common cold, influenza, malignant pleurisy, low fevers, agues, indigestion and weakness in general, being managed as above directed, according to the effect desired."

American fields and forests proved to be a rich source of new drug plants and substitutes for foreign products.

The bark of beautiful flowering dogwood (*Cornus florida*) was used as a substitute for Peruvian bark (*Cinchona* or quinine). The bark of kinnikinnik or swamp dogwood (*Cornus amomum*) was also used and believed by some to be preferable to flowering dogwood.

Indian doctors believed the American ipecacs (*Euphorbia ipecacuanha* or *E. corollata*) superior to the imported article.

American cascara sagrada is considered by many far superior to the Chinese rhubarb that was so long used for chronic constipation. The roots of native mandrake or mayapple (*Podophyllum peltatum*) are powerfully cathartic. Indians ate the delicious fruit and made an insect poison of its leaves. Our yellow-flowering American senna bush (*Cassia marilandica*) has laxative properties similar to the Egyptian senna. Balmony or turtlehead (*Chelone glabra*); Culver's root (*Leptandra virginica*); bark of the root of Indian physic (*Gillenia trifoliata*); and butternut (*Juglens cinera*) also served as cathartics. Jacob Bigelow, M.D., wrote in 1818: "The inner bark of the butternut tree, especially that obtained from the root, affords one of the most mild and efficacious laxatives which we possess. . . . During the revolutionary war, when foreign medicines were scarce, this extract was resorted to by many of the army surgeons, as a substitute for more expensive imported drugs. In dysentery it seems at one time to have acquired a sort of specific reputation."

The finest demulcent and emollient in the botanical kingdom is derived from the inner bark of the American species of elm (*Ulmus fulva*).

Native artemisia, aromatic bitter herbs, were plentiful over a wide range of the New World. Cooling herbs, such as varieties of pennyroyals (*Hedeoma*), mountain mints (*Koellia*), and camphoraceous species of monarda were common in American fields. Sassafras bark of root; twigs, bark and berries of spice bush (*Benzoin aestivale*); roots of wild ginger (*Asarum canadense*); anise-flavored roots of sweet cicelys (*Washingtonia claytoni* and *W. longistylis*); vanilla-scented deer's tongue (*Liatris odoratissima*); fiery leaves of smartweed (*Polygonum punctatum*); the hot chili-flavored roots of yerba mansa (*Anemopsis californica*); the biting corms of Indian turnips (*Arisaema triphyllum*); the acrid bloodroot (*Sanguinaria canadensis*); and innumerable other native plants were utilized in folk medication.

Nature appears to have been most prolific in its supply of blood-staunching plants wherever man immigrated in the vegetable kingdom. One of the most effective native plants was Canada fleabane or blood-staunch (*Erigeron canadensis*)—a common unattractive weed respected by all that were familiar with its virtues. The roots of wild alum or cranesbill (*Geranium maculatum*) were also a godsend for Indians and white men on dire occasions in the wilderness. An 1802 record stated, "Wild alum is one of the greatest vulneraries and astringents of the vegetable creation, and highly extolled for its styptic power in hemorrhages of every description. These properties have been sufficiently ascertained by experience." Perhaps the most widely used of all astringents is that made from our native witch hazel bush (*Hamamelis virginiana*).

Many plants brought from Europe and other sources have become a part of American flora and grow vigorously in the soils of the New World. Catnip, feverfew, costmary, hound's tongue, elecampane, celandine, comfrey, coltsfoot, wormwood, mugwort, hollyhock and others grown by colonists, still linger near old settlements or farms where homes stood long ago. Old garden medicinals, burdock, curled dock, sour dock, couch grass, wild carrot, yarrow, selfheal and others remain unyieldingly in gardens and farms, thriving in competition with the toughest native wild plants. Indians once dubbed common plantain "white man's footsteps" because the plant appeared to grow wherever the white men trod. Plantain is perfectly at home in the white man's lawn with dandelion, ground ivy, sorrel and other old-time foreign folk-medicinals. Bouncing bet, the soap plant of colonial times; the lovely blue-flowering chicory; the golden-flowered tansy and the St. John's wort of the Old World are now familiar wayside weeds over much of the United States.

Spices, molasses, sugar, etc., were brought to frontier settlements by itinerant peddlers. Folks living in isolated wilderness used honey and maple sugar when available. According to Millspaugh, the sap of the butternut tree also was boiled in early spring to make "a fine sugar equal, if not superior, to that of the maple." Barley and Indian meals, potatoes, carrots, turnips, cucumbers, onions, garlic and other garden crops also served as folk materia medica.

Pioneers living in Indian territories had to rely on wild animals for survival. Fats and oils of raccoon, skunk, snake, deer, etc., were medicinal substitutions for mutton tallow, butter, lard, chicken fat, goose grease, etc. The oil of bear was especially highly regarded by settlers as well as the Indians. It was often referred to as "soft oil" in folk literature. The Indian herb doctor, Monroe, author (1824) and recorder of a large number of Indian discoveries in the medical art that were never before published, stated: "Bear oil is less cloying than that of any other animal. It is used to advantage by Indian women for a considerable time before delivery. It is likewise of great service in phthisica, quinsy, stiff joints, etc."

Native trees proved a rich source of useful gums and resins. Monroe lists pine tar as "a thick, black resinous juice, melted by fire out of old pine and fir trees, and is good in plasters. A water is obtained by putting a pint of tar into a gallon of water, well warmed and stirred, then settled and poured off for use. It is good in debilities in old age and cancer humors."

Vinegar is a folk medicinal from the Old World. It has been long used diluted with water as a refreshing drink to allay thirst and diminish excessive heat in fevers. It was used as an astringent in hemorrhages from the nose, lungs, stomach and uterus. Vinegar was much used as a gargle and a cooling wash for burns, itching skin, poison oak and ivy. Pierpont Bowker wrote in 1836, "The juice of the leaves of marigold (*Calendula*) mixed with vinegar, and used as a bath, will ease hot swellings." Impregnated with aromatic herbs, gums or oils, vinegar was sprinkled on the floors of sick chambers to cover unpleasant odors. It was formerly regarded as a stimulant, disinfectant and antiseptic.

Wines and liquors were also much used in folk medication when available. Like aromatic teas, wines were often taken with pulverized botanicals that could not be boiled in water. Wines, such as port, sherry and madeira, were used with recipes for female weakness and general debility. Gin was considered a good diuretic and was used in old-time dropsical formulae. Brandy and whiskey were regarded as stimulants and restoratives and were the bases for countless recipes for bitters. Hot toddy made with bourbon was a standard remedy at the first sign of sniffles. Rum was commonly used in concoctions for coughs, catarrh and rheumatism.

Chemicals used in folk medicine consisted of such simple materials as salt, sulphur and lime, items which were readily available in the kitchen and on the farm. Mineral salts were obtained by reducing certain woods and plants to ashes. In dire conditions inventive pioneers found suitable substitutes for most of their needs.

OLD PLANT NAMES, WORDS AND PHRASES

Many early American popular medical publications, especially the small books printed by the Indian herb or root doctors, described the medicinal uses of native plants that were known only by the vernacular names given them by the settlers and Indians. Linnaeus's Latin classification of plants was still unknown to most people of the New World as many species were still in the process of being classified. Native plants were known better for their uses or for some conspicuous feature. Ague weed (*Eupatorium perfoliatum*) was much used for a common complaint suffered among settlers who lived in damp log cabins that often had earth floors and no glass windows. There were also ague bark (*Ptelea trifoliata*), ague grass (*Aletris farinosa*) and other plants for ague. *Aletris farinosa* was also known as maiden's relief because a decoction made of the roots was used to ease menstrual periods. Other popular frontier medicines were sore throat root (*Caulophyllum thalictroides*), sweat root (*Polemonium reptans*), emetic weed (*Lobelia inflata*), backache root (*Liatris spicata*), bellyache weed (*Solidago bicolor*), convulsion weed or fitroot (*Monotropa uniflora*), pleurisy root (*Asclepias tuberosa*), coughwort (*Trillium cernuum*), cut-heal (*Geum rivale*), cancer weed (*Salvia lyrata*), rheumatism weed (*Chimphila maculata*), mouth root, (*Coptis trifolia*), canker root (*Statice caroliniana*), etc. Walpole tea or New Jersey tea (*Ceanothus americanus*), Carolina tea or Indian black drink (*Ilex vomitoria*), and Oswego tea (*Monarda didyma*) are representative of a few native beverage plants.

Because of their very high silicon content, varieties of horsetail grasses (*Equisetum*) were used to polish pewter, so the plants were known as pewterwort. Dye weed was a common name for *Hydrastis canadensis* because its golden roots were used by the Indians for dyeing deer hides. The majority of our native plants have one or more common names that have tenaciously remained with the plants since pioneer times. The vernacular names of plants are very confusing because they often refer to entirely different species. Dye weed, for example, can mean dozens of plants used for that purpose. Much of this confusion has been clarified by authoritative botanists. Charles F. Millspaugh's three volumes, *American Medicinal Plants* (1887), is a notable example where identifications of important native medicinal plants have been established.

Until recent years, with the exception of educational centers and people fortunate enough to have been able to attend schools, English-American words and phrases were loosely used by the majority of Americans. Diseases were referred to broadly as humors, troubles, disorders, obstructions, complaints and inflammations. Canker often referred to an infection, ulcerous sore or malignant disease. Cholics referred to intestinal pains of any kind. Terms such as sure cure, infallible cure, sovereign remedy, all or any disease, etc., were used indiscriminately in folk-medical literature. People were not concerned with the work of Linnaeus nor with the precise definition of words in Noah Webster's *American Dictionary of the English Language* (1828). Americans—a conglomeration of many nationalities moving westward—were more interested in carrying seeds, farm tools and guns for their protection in the new lands. If books accompanied the pioneers, they were invariably Bibles or small pocket-size medical books to help them where there were no doctors.

Common Conditions Treated in American Folk Practice

ASTHMA   31

    Sirups for asthmatic cough   33
    Smoke mixtures to ease difficult breathing   34

BED WETTING   36

BILIOUS COMPLAINTS   36

BITES and STINGS of INSECTS   38

    Bee or wasp stings   38
    Spider bites   39
    Miscellaneous bites   39

BLOOD CONDITIONS   40

    Blood purifiers   40
    Blood "thinners"   42

BOILS   42

    Alleged preventives   44

BOWEL COMPLAINTS   45

    Bowels inflamed   45
    External applications   46

BREASTS   46

    To develop   46
    To increase milk   46
    To dry up breasts   47
    Sore, swelled, hard or caked breasts   47
    Salves for sore breasts   48

Inflamed breasts 49
Sore nipples 49

BRONCHITIS 50

BURNS and SCALDS 51
Salves and oils used 55

CARBUNCLES 57

CATARRH 58
Mixtures for snuffs and smoking 58
Chronic catarrh 59
Catarrh in children 59
Catarrh in lungs 59
Catarrh in stomach 59
Catarrh in bladder 59

CHICKEN POX 60

CHILBLAINS 60

CHILLS 63

CHOKING or SWALLOWING
FOREIGN SUBSTANCE 63

COLDS 64
Chest colds 67
Head colds 67
Head colds in children and infants 68

COLIC 68
External applications 71

CONSTIPATION 71
Constipation in infants and children 75

CONVULSIONS 75

COUGHS 76
Dry cough 84

CROUP 84

DEBILITY 87
Debility of the aged 88

DIARRHEA	89
Infants and children	89
Older children and adults	90
Chronic diarrhea	93
Diet during diarrhea	94
DYSENTERY	94
Chronic dysentery	99
EARS	100
Earache	100
Removing foreign substance from ear	101
Removing insects from ear	102
Deafness caused by wax accumulation	102
Deficiency of wax	103
Running ears	104
ECZEMA	104
Internal and external treatments	106
ERYSIPELAS or ST. ANTHONY'S FIRE	107
EYES	109
Inflamed, irritated or sore	109
Eyewashes	111
Black or bruised eye	112
Foreign matter in the eye	112
Sties	112
Weak eyes	113
Weeping eyes	114
FAINT	115
FATIGUE	116
FEET	116
Athlete's foot	116
Bunions	116
Cold feet	116
Corns	117
Ingrown toenails	119
Itching feet	119
Perspiring feet	119
Swollen feet	119
Tender and aching feet	120

FELON or WHITLOW 120

FEMALE WEAKNESS 123

FEVERS 125

    Ague, malarial, intermittent fever 125
    External applications for chills of fever 128
    Drinks for fever 129
    Alleged fever preventives 130

FEVER SORES 131

FLU, INFLUENZA, GRIPPE 131

    Asiatic flu 133
    Convalescing after flu 133
    Cough after flu 133

FROSTBITE 133

    Frozen feet 134

HAYFEVER 135

HEADACHES 136

    Bilious headache 136
    Dissipation, mental exhaustion or menstrual
        period 136
    Nervous headache 136
    Sick headache 137
    External applications 138

HICCUP or HICCOUGH 139

HIVES or NETTLE RASH 141

    External applications 142

HYPOCHONDRIA 142

HYSTERIA 142

    Alleged preventives 143

INSOMNIA 144

    Recipes for infants and children 146

INTOXICATION 146

ITCH 148

    Internal medicine for itch 149

JAUNDICE   150

KIDNEYS   153

    To promote urine   153
    Too free, or no control of urine   156
    Chronic kidney complaint   157
    Scalding urine, or irritation in absence
        of systemic or organic disease   157
    Inflammation. Palliatives for
        nephritic paroxysms   158
    Pus in urine   160
    Blood in urine   160
    Gravel and stones. Attempted treatments   161

LEUCORRHEA   164

    Douches   165

LIGHTNING   165

LIVER   166

    To relieve distress   166
    Chronic liver complaint   168

MEASLES   170

MENSES   171

    Suppressed, obstructed, scanty   171
    Painful, difficult menses; cramps   173
    Profuse, excessive   174
    Regulators (folk term)   175
    Change of life (menopause)   176

MOUTH   177

    Bad breath   177
    Canker or thrush   177
    Miscellaneous mouth complaints   180
    Gums   180
    Lips   180

MUMPS   181

MUSCULAR CRAMPS   182

NAUSEA   184

    Sea or car sickness   184

NERVOUSNESS 184

NEURALGIA 185

    External applications 186

NIGHT SWEATS 187

NOSE 188

    Nosebleed 188
    Obstructions in the nose 189

PAIN 190

    External applications 190
    External and internal 191

PHLEGM 191

PILES or HEMORRHOIDS 192

PLASTERS 197

PLEURISY 197

POISON IVY, POISON OAK, etc. 198

POULTICES 200

PREGNANCY 205

    To facilitate childbirth 205
    To prevent abortion or miscarriage 207
    Nausea or sick stomach 208
    Constipation 208
    To relieve scalding and itching caused by urine 209
    Cramps 209
    Convulsions 209
    Swelling of feet and limbs 209
    Distention of skin 209
    Afterpains 210
    Discharges after childbirth 210

RHEUMATISM 212

    Internal and external medication 217
    External applications and methods used to
        palliate pains of rheumatism 218
    Sciatic rheumatism 220

RINGWORM 220

SCALL HEAD 222

SCROFULA 223
    Salves for scrofulous skin disease 223

SCURVY 224

SKIN 224
    Chafed skin 224
    Chapped hands 224
    Freckles 225
    Fungus 225
    Impetigo 226
    Pimples 226
    Prickly heat 226
    Rash 227
    Scars 227
    Sunburn 228

SLIVERS or SPLINTERS 228

SORES and SURFACE ULCERS 228

SPRAINS 231

STIFFNESS 233
    Neck 233
    Joints 233

STOMACH DISTRESS 234
    Acidity, heartburn or sour stomach 234
    Flatulence or gas 235
    Cramps caused by flatulence or gas 235
    Indigestion or dyspepsia 237
    Nervous, upset or strained stomach 241
    Weak or sick stomach 241
    Inflamed stomach, to temporarily allay irritation 243
    Palliatives for gastric ulcer 243

SWELLINGS in EARLY STAGES 243
    White or hard swellings 243
    Soft, flabby swellings 244
    Swollen limbs 244

TEETH   245

    Cleaning and preventing decay   245
    Toothache   246
    Bleeding from extraction   248
    Teething infants   248
    Cleaning infants' teeth   249

THROAT   249

    Simple sore throat   249
    Tonsillitis or quinsy   251
    External applications   252
    Hoarseness   253
    Throat tickle   255

TONICS and BITTERS   255

    Spring tonics   257
    Spring tonics for ladies and children   259

VOMITING   260

WARTS   263

WEIGHT   264

    For thin and scrawny children   264
    To reduce weight of adults   264

WEN   265

WHOOPING COUGH   266

    Recipes used to alleviate the
        paroxysms and alleged cures   266
    External applications   267

WORMS   268

    Pinworms   270
    Tapeworms   271

WOUNDS   271

    Bruises   273
    To prevent skin discoloring after bruises 274
    Cuts   275
    Excessive bleeding   276
    Nail wounds   278

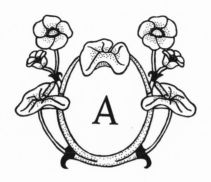

ASTHMA

Get a muskrat skin and wear it over the lungs, with the fur side next to the body. It will bring certain relief.

Miss E. Neill, 1890

Sniff a pinch of borax up the nostrils each morning and clear after a minute.

The oil of goose is a good remedy but the feathers are very hurtful to those who lie upon them.

J. Monroe, 1824

Take 3 egg shells, roast them brown, and pound them up coarsely; mix these with ½ pint molasses, take a spoon 3 times a day. The cure is effectual in common cases.

P. F. Bowker, 1836

It is said that the juice of radishes is good for dry or convulsive asthma. A small dose of castor oil taken occasionally, will be found beneficial; or new milk drunk morning and evening.

The American Family Receipt Book, 1854

Sleep on a pillow made of dried elder leaves. It will give complete relief for hayfever or asthma.

When the symptoms appear, at once place the feet in warm water, and take a decoction of catnip herb or pennyroyal herb, to produce a gentle perspiration. If the attack continues, take a tablespoon of the tincture of lobelia in a cup of warm tea, every ½ hour. The following remedy has produced marked results in severe cases: Take ½ ounce of well-bruised seneca snakeroot; immerse in 1 pint of water, and boil over a slow fire till reduced to ½ pint. Dose, a tablespoon every 10 to 15 minutes. A teaspoon of mustard seed, taken in tea or soup, morning and evening, has cured many cases.

Asthma weed is a grand article to be relied upon for the alleviation or cure. It may be given in ½ or whole teaspoon doses of the pulverized seeds or leaves and pods, at bed time, or when the fits are coming on, and at any other time when urgency of the symptoms appears to require it.

H. Howard, 1857

Beat, in a mortar, equal quantities of the leaves of hedge mustard and virgin honey, so as to make a thin conserve. This may be taken quite at discretion, according to the state of the disease, and the benefit experienced. Hedge mustard, both seed and herb, is medicinally considered as warm, dry, attentuating, opening, and expectorant. It is vulnerary, causes plentiful spitting, and renders breathing easier.

Take 1 or 2 pieces of *Aloe vera* leaves sliced crosswise; steep in cold water for an hour. Strain off aloe and drink the water several times a day.

Take 4 ounces of wild white daisy blossoms and pour over them 1 pint of boiling water. Steep 1 hour and strain. Dose: 1 tablespoon 3 times a day.

Wild plum bark was highly regarded in folk medicine. Boil ½ ounce of the inner bark in 1 pint of water for 15 or 20 minutes. Strain when cool. Dose: 1 or 2 wineglassfuls a day.

An ounce of the powder of blood root steeped in 1 quart of gin or whiskey, and a tablespoon taken every morning, is good for those who are troubled with asthma.

Take 1 ounce of skunk cabbage root, 5 ounces rock candy; steep in 3 cups of boiling water. Allow to stand 7 to 14 days. Strain. Add equal amount of whiskey. Take shot glassful.

Take 4 ounces of hen's fat, and with it simmer a little of the root of skunk cabbage. Dose: 1 teaspoon, 3 times a day.

Dr. A. A. Benezet, 1826

Take a seed bowl of a skunk cabbage, that grows close to the ground, at the bottom of the leaves. Cut it up fine, stew this in 4 ounces of hen's fat till it is dry. Strain it off, take teaspoon 3 times a day. Make a syrup of queen-of-the-meadow root, and white swamp honeysuckle blossoms. Sweeten this with honey, add to a quart of syrup half a pint of brandy. Rarely fails.

Cut an ounce stick of licorice into slices. Steep this in a quart of water 24 hours, and use it, when you are worse than usual, as common drink.

Take powdered licorice, powdered elecampane, powdered aniseed of each 1 teaspoon. Add 10 grains powdered ipecac, 10 grains powdered lobelia, and enough pine tar to form into pills of ordinary size. Take 3 or 4 pills on going to bed. Excellent for shortness of breath.

Mrs. M. W. Ellsworth, 1897

Take ¼ ounce powdered elecampane root; ½ ounce powdered licorice; as much flower of sulphur and powdered aniseed, and 2 ounces of rock candy powdered. Make all into pills, with sufficient quantity of tar. Take 4 large pills when going to rest. This is an incomparable medicine.

Phthisic in children. Take 2 ounces of licorice stick, of parsley root 4 ounces; spikenard root 4 ounces; snakeroot 4 ounces; boil them well in 4 quarts of water. After it is strained, sweeten with loaf sugar, or honey. Dose, a glass night and morning.

Take ½ ounce each of licorice root, mullein leaves, hoarhound herb, lungwort herb, and sage. Boil in 1 quart of water for 20 minutes. Strain when cool. Take wineglassful at bedtime.

Other botanicals that have been used for asthma: Gum plant, Ephedra species, Hungarian wormwood [*Artemisia pontica*], false saffron [*Carthamus tinctorius*], true saffron [*Crocus sativus*], thyme herb.

SIRUPS FOR ASTHMATIC COUGH

Take 1 teaspoon of hot honey every ¼ hour. It will relieve severe spasms of asthma.

Boil 1 ounce of asthma-weed in 3 cups of water. Boil until dark red, and add a cup of cane sugar. Boil down to 2 cups. Take 2 teaspoons every 10 to 15 minutes until relieved.

Take ½ ounce each of asthma-weed, scullcap herb, and lady slipper root. Boil for 10 minutes in 1 pint of water. Allow to stand until cool then strain off botanicals. Add a little ginger and enough honey to make a syrup. Take tablespoon 3 or 4 times a day.

Take 2 ounces of elecampane root, 2 ounces sweet-flag root, 2 ounces spikenard, and 2 ounces of common chalk; beat them in a mortar, till they become very fine, then add 1 pound of honey, and beat them all together. Take teaspoon 3 times a day.

Take ½ ounce each of flaxseed, licorice, boneset herb, and slippery elm. Simmer together in 1 pint of water, strain, add ½ pint of best molasses and ¼ pound of loaf sugar. Simmer all together. After it has cooled, bottle it tightly.

A strong tea made of the bark of the root of common mullein and sweetened to the consistency of syrup, of which 4 teaspoons are given to a child as a dose, and frequently repeated.

Take ½ pint of the juice of stinging nettles; boil and scum it, and mix it up with as much clarified honey. Take a spoonful morning and evening.

A spoonful of mustard seed mixed with molasses, taken several times a day, is good for asthma.

Take 1 pound of sliced garlic, and 1 quart of boiling water, and let it soak for 10 or 12 hours, keeping the water warm all the while. Then strain off, add 4 pounds of double refined sugar, and bottle it up. This is an excellent syrup, and may be used to advantage. A teaspoon is a dose, when you feel like coughing.

SMOKE MIXTURES TO EASE DIFFICULT BREATHING

The dried leaves of jimson weed smoked with tobacco will relieve asthma. Care should be taken in doing this, and the results closely observed, that the effect may not be too severe.

Another recipe advises a few aniseeds mixed with jimson weed leaves.

Mix a little rosemary herb with jimson weed leaves to prevent nausea. Smoke a pipeful in the evening before going to bed. The practice should be continued for some time.

Gather the green leaves of the jimson weed, after the plant blossoms, and dry them in the shade. When dry, soak a few hours in a strong solution of purified niter, common saltpeter does not answer, 3 ounces to 1 pint soft water. Powder the niter finely, and pour on hot water to dissolve it. Soak the dried leaves in this solution, redry in the shade, then pulverize the leaves and keep from the air in box or bottle. Put a rounding teaspoon of the nitrated powder on a plate, and touch a lighted match to the heap, when, if properly done, it burns without a blaze, throwing off considerable smoke. Breathe the smoke arising from it and inhale as much as you can of the fumes. It will cause some coughing at first, but this helps to clear the throat and bronchial tubes of phlegm, and soon subsides and gives great relief.

Mrs. M. W. Ellsworth, 1897

Take 4 ounces jimson weed leaves, 4 ounces skunk cabbage leaves, 2 ounces coltsfoot leaves, 2 ounces lobelia herb. Rub to a coarse powder. Mix, and dissolve 2 ounces of nitrate of potassia, in ½ pint water; mix well with powder; dry thoroughly, smoke in ordinary clay pipe morning and evening.

Smoke crushed cubebs in a pipe, emitting the smoke through the nose. If the nose is stopped up so that it is almost impossible to breathe, one pipeful usually will clear the head. After smoking, do not expose yourself to cold air for at least 15 minutes.

Take the dried leaves of rosemary, shred small, and smoke them in a tobacco pipe. It will help those that have a cough or phthisic, or consumption, by warming and drying the thin distillations which cause those diseases.

Smoke in a clay pipe a mixture made of 2 parts chamomile flowers, 1 part mullein leaves and a small part cloves or cubeb berries.

The dried leaves of mullein may be smoked like tobacco to relieve nasal catarrh and asthma.

Smoke the leaves of eucalyptus tree.

The dried bark of green ozier smoked, relieves the asthma—the aborigines smoke it as a substitute for tobacco.

BED WETTING

A teaspoon of honey given just before bedtime will help the retention of water.

Steep tablespoon of the herb and flowers of St. John's wort in 1 cup of boiling water and allow to stand 20 minutes. Strain and sweeten. Give 1 or 2 cups daily to child until cured.

Take 1 ounce of mullein herb to 1 pint of boiling water. Steep 10 minutes. Strain. Dose, 1 wineglassful night and morning.

Take good red bark 2 ounces, 1 quart of wine, steep the bark in the wine 24 hours; let the patient drink a tablespoon, if 2 or 3 years old; if older, a little more at a time.

BILIOUS COMPLAINTS

Also see LIVER.

Pour a cup of boiling water on a tablespoon of boneset and let it stand until cold. Strain. Take a small swallow occasionally.

When the person is attacked with bilious colic, give an injection of boneset, and let the patient drink freely of the same herb. If this should not effect a cure, give an injection of tobacco leaves, boiled strong, and afterwards a sirup of the buckthorn, which will seldom fail of effecting a cure.

Boneset herb 2 ounces; senna leaves 1 ounce; water 1 pint. Mix and boil. To 1 pint of this decoction, add ½ tablespoon salt, ½ pint molasses, 1 tablespoon compound tincture of lobelia and capsicum. Give the whole warm, for enema, and repeat every 10 or 15 minutes until bowels are emptied.

Slice some green walnuts and leave them digest 1 or 2 weeks in enough whiskey or alcohol to cover them. Dose, a teaspoon every ½ hour, till relief is obtained.

Take of white walnut bark, elder bark, and dogwood bark, each a handful; boil them in 4 quarts of water down to 1 quart; strain, and add ½ tablespoon of saltpeter. Dose, a teaspoon or 2, 3 or 4 times a day. This has given relief, and also broken up the disposition of bilious colic, where everything else has failed.

Boil ½ ounce of colic root in 1 pint of water 3 or 4 minutes. Strain when cool. Drink ½ teacupful every ½ hour till relief is obtained.

One pound of common milkweed root, green, or ½ pound of dry; pound it, boil it in 1 quart of water down to ½ pint. Take ½ of it at a dose. But if a person should be taken violently, dig roots enough to fill a pint basin, pound it and pour on boiling water so as to get the strength. Strain and drink it as soon as you can, and it will cure when nothing else will.

Take dandelion root and poplar tree bark, each ½ pound; steep out all the strength; simmer it down thick; add molasses, and take 1 teaspoon 4 times a day; or, take ¼ pound of black cherry tree bark, 1 ounce of bloodroot; steep in 1½ pints of brandy for 3 days; then add 1 gill of water, and 1 gill of molasses; let it steep 3 days and it is fit for use. Dose, from 1 tablespoon to ½ wineglassful 2 or 3 times a day. If it should brace the stomach too much, take less, if not, take a little more.

Anti-bilious powder. Take of pearlash 4 parts; white and red birthroot, 1 part; pulverize and mix—put them into a tight bottle for use. Put a teaspoon of this mixture in a cup and pour on a gill of weak vinegar, or vinegar and sour cider mixed—to be taken while in the act of effervescence. Repeat it every 5 minutes, until it gives relief.

BITES and STINGS of INSECTS

Bees leave their stingers in the skin and they must be removed first. Wasps do not leave stingers.

BEE OR WASP STINGS

For bee or wasp sting apply honey.

When far from usual remedies, clap a handful of damp dirt or moist clay on the wound, removing when dry and heated and replacing with fresh application.

Simple remedies for bee and insect stings are a piece of raw beef, a strong solution of ammonia, vinegar and salt, or borax moistened with lemon juice, or tincture of myrrh.

A little lemon juice applied to a sting or insect bite will soon relieve the pain.

If bee sting looks fiery and swells, poultice it with cloth or cotton wool damped with lime water or a strong solution of bicarbonate of soda.

Apply a strong decoction of wild chamomile flowers.

Make a strong decoction of *Lobelia inflata* and apply it often. An infallible cure.

Olive oil or sweet oil affords relief from stings of bees or other insects.

Castor oil is said to be an infallible remedy for the stings of bees and other insects. It appears to counteract the poison and allay the pain as soon as applied.

Kerosene often relieves the pain of stings at once and prevents swelling.

An application of snuff on yellow jacket or hornet bites usually is very effective.

Apply damp tea leaves to wasp stings.

Rub wasp stings with clove of garlic, sliced onion or raw potato.

Apply some good rubbing alcohol on cotton for wasp stings.

SPIDER BITES

Apply vinegar, ammonia or tobacco juice.

Take alum powder and white of an egg beaten and make a small poultice. Apply to the part and it will take out swelling and relieve the pain.

When stung by an insect or bitten by a spider, suck the wound vigorously for a moment, and then cover it with a cloth wet with quite strong ammonia. A mixture of equal parts of common baking soda and salt well rubbed into the wound will often give relief.

The expressed juice of the common plantain leaves is an effectual antidote to the bite of venomous spiders. Apply some of the juice to the wound, and take about a gill of it internally; or chew the leaves.

It was recorded in a Virginia paper, that a gentleman was bitten above the knee by a spider. A few minutes after, he perceived a pain shooting upwards from the spot which soon reached his heart. A quantity of plantain was immediately gathered and bruised, and the juice squeezed out and swallowed, which stopped the progress of the poison, so that a cure of the bite was obtained immediately.

Elias Smith, Physician, 1826

MISCELLANEOUS BITES

Ant bites, apply eau de Cologne.

Centipede or scorpion bites, apply ammonia.

Chigger bites, use butter thickened with salt.

Horsefly bites, apply ammonia.

BLOOD CONDITIONS

BLOOD PURIFIERS

(An old term still in popular use in folk medicine, as well as in many modern foreign herbals.)

The bark of prickly ash, particularly the bark of the roots is highly esteemed by the natives for its medicinal qualities. There is no doubt but that the decoction of it will expeditiously and radically remove all impurities of the blood.

J. Carver, 1779

Instead of water, drink several times a day a decoction made of sycamore root.

Letter, 1914

Make an infusion of the leaves of sweet fern. Drink a cupful several times a day.

Figwort herb surely is a fine remedy for cleansing the blood of a lot of impurities.

J. K. F.

One ounce yellow dock root, ½ ounce horseradish root in 1 quart of hard cider. Allow to steep at least a week. Drink a wineglassful 4 times a day.

The infusion of the herb and root of cold-water-root purifies the blood and juices, and prevents fevers if administered in season.

Drink freely of an infusion made with boiling water and spicewood twigs.

The juice of common beet root is purifying to the blood and juices: but after the juice is boiled out, they are hard to digest, and afford but little nourishment.

Black cohosh root is a powerful stimulant. It purges the blood and humors, and removes swellings and rheumatism. It may be used in removing obstructions of the system. A teaspoon of the powder of the root, in a gill of hot water, is a sufficient dose.

Take 1 pound spikenard root, 1 pound sarsaparilla root, 1 pound bull thistle root, 1 pound yellow dock root, ½ pound celandine herb, 1 pound red clover flowers, ½ pound dandelion root, ½ pound queen-of-the-meadow tops, ½ pound elder bark of root, ¼ pound sweet apple tree bark of root. Boil in 3 gallons of water, and boil until reduced to 1 gallon. Strain when cool, add 1 pint molasses, and 1 pint gin, ½ ounce oil of wintergreen. Keep in cool place. Dose, a wineglassful 3 times a day.

Take equal parts of American sarsaparilla, yellow dock root, stillingia root, elder flowers, and black haw bark. Mix well. Use tablespoon to each cupful of water. Boil 10 minutes. Strain when cool. Take 2 cupfuls a day in small doses.

Dandelion and sarsaparilla, each 1 drachm of dried root. Put into a pitcher and pour over it 1 pint of boiling water at night. Drink the next day at intervals. Do this 1 month, the effect will be very good.

Take 6 teaspoons black alder bark, 2 of burdock root, 2 of yellow dock root, 2 of sarsaparilla, 2 of red clover flowers, 3 of licorice root and 1 of coriander seeds. Mix well. Add 1 tablespoon to a cupful of water and boil 5 minutes. Strain when cool. Dose, ½ cupful 2 or 3 times daily.

Boil 1 ounce burdock root in 1 pint of water for 10 minutes. Strain when cool. Take tablespoon 3 or 4 times daily. May be taken with a little molasses.

Take ½ ounce each of coneflower root, yellow dock root and burdock root. Simmer for 15 minutes in 1 quart of water. Strain when cool. Drink wineglassful 2 or 3 times daily.

Take white ash bark, white poplar bark, burdock root and black cherry bark, simmer them together, and make a constant drink of it, and it will cleanse the blood, and cure tumors on the body.

Take 6 fair size roots of each of the following: dandelion, burdock, and yellow dock. Clean as you would carrots. Take 1 cup of inner bark from wild black cherry (removing all dark bark). Add the botanicals to ½ gallon water and stew it till it is about ⅓ left. Strain through fine cloth several times until it is clear. Add a preservative. One teaspoon is sufficient twice daily.

Take the inner bark of wild cherry, bark of sassafras root and the root of burdock, equal parts. Mix. Boil a tablespoon in 1 pint of water for 5 minutes. Steep until cold. Strain. Drink 1 cupful daily.

Take ½ ounce each of burdock root and sassafras bark of root. Boil for 15 minutes in 1 pint of water. Strain when cool. Dose, wineglassful 2 or 3 times a day.

Take ½ ounce each of sassafras root, fumitory herb, figwort herb and blue-flag root. Boil in 2 quarts of water for 20 minutes. Dose, ½ teacupful 3 or 4 times daily after meals.

Make a decoction of equal parts of sassafras and sarsaparilla. Drink wineglassful 2 or 3 times daily.

Take a gallon of inner bark of white beech, a large handful of blackberry root and also of sassafras root. Cover with boiling water and strain when lukewarm. Add 1 pint baker's yeast and 1 cup sugar. Let it stand 24 hours in a warm place. Strain and set in a cool place. Take a wineglassful before meals.

BLOOD "THINNERS"

Heart's ease has a tendency to thin the blood.

Yarrow will cause a brisk circulation of the blood.

Drink freely, with or without meals, infusion made with the bark of root of sassafras.

BOILS

Also see POULTICES.

The skin of a boiled egg is the most efficacious remedy that can be applied to a boil. Peel it carefully, wet and apply to the part affected. It will draw off the matter, and relieve the soreness in a few hours.

Miss E. Neill, 1890

A poultice made with thin slices of salt pork put between clean, white cloths is good for boils. Change 2 or 3 times a day, until the boil has been drawn to a head.

Make a poultice of 1 cup of milk and 3 teaspoons of salt. Heat milk, add salt gradually so it will not curdle; cook until smooth and creamy, then add enough flour to thicken. Divide this into 4 poultices and apply in succession every ½ hour. This will remove the soreness and it should be kept oiled until healed.

Cut a red onion crosswise, scoop out a little from one piece and place the cup over the boil. It will draw.

Bathe frequently with strong vinegar and apply poultice made with mashed leaves of snapbean.

Stir 1 teaspoon powdered alum in 1 pint of warm water. Use as wet poultice to make boils come to a head.

Mrs. S. C. W.

A poultice of ripe figs is one of the best things known for carbuncles or boils. Figs must be well washed and peeled.

The application [poultice] of the leaves of common garden cabbage, or of skunk cabbage, to the part, will have a tendency to produce moisture of the skin, arrest inflammation, and dissolve the tumor.

The leaves of dollar-vine were used as a poultice to draw out boils. The leaves also were cooked with cornmeal for this purpose.

Kentucky recipe

Boils or risings are best relieved by the application of a poultice of mashed elderberry leaves.

Make a poultice of equal parts of beech bark with wheat bran and apply as hot as can be borne.

Boils should be brought to a head by warm poultices of chamomile flowers, or boiled white lily root, or onion root, by fermentation with hot water, or by stimulating plasters. When ripe they should be destroyed by a needle or lancet. But this should not be attempted until they are thoroughly proved.

Apply a poultice of the mashed fresh blades of sea squill.

Make a poultice of equal parts of ground ivy, yarrow and chamomile flowers. Steep mixture in boiling water until botanicals are completely softened. Strain off the liquid and apply mash to boil. Keep poultice bandage moist with the strained-off decoction.

Black horehound herb applied as a poultice will mollify angry boils.

Mix a good pinch of shredded slippery elm to boiling water until a stiff paste is formed. Apply directly to the boil. This poultice must be repeated every hour until suppuration sets in and then every 2 hours till the discharge has ceased.

When boils are coming to a head, and are very painful, apply a poultice of equal parts of slippery elm bark, in powder, and lobelia leaves; or a bread and milk poultice, to which powdered lobelia has been added.

After the boil has opened, wash it twice a day with Castile soapsuds, to which some whisky has been added, and if necessary, apply a poultice of powdered slippery elm a tablespoonful, ginger a teaspoon, powdered bloodroot as much as will lie on a dime, water enough to form a poultice.

J. King, M.D., 1855

ALLEGED PREVENTIVES

Make a strong decoction of equal parts of burdock root and sassafras. Drink ½ cupful at a time, several a day.

When persons are subject to boils, they may break up the tendency to them by drinking rather freely of an infusion of burdock seed, sassafras bark, and St. John's wort, equal parts of each.

For a person who has boils grate 1 teaspoon nutmeg and once a day swallow this on some food such as custards or puddings and you won't have any more boils.

Boil 1 ounce of *Echinacea angustifolia* root in 1 pint of water. Dose, take wineglass twice daily, and also dab a little of the decoction on the affected parts.

Procure 1 ounce horseradish roots, 1 ounce yellow dock root, 1 quart of cider. Boil 10 minutes. Drink a wineglassful 3 times a day.

Take a handful of inner bark of the birch tree, and boil in a pint of water. Take a wineglassful each morning.

N. M., 1931

Steep a handful of boneset herb in a quart jar full of cold water. Allow to stand overnight. Drink the water instead of plain water.

BOWEL COMPLAINTS

An infusion made with red raspberry leaves is excellent for children when bowels are loose and while teething.

Mrs. A. Matteson, 1894

The dried leaves of peach tree prepared as a tea is very useful in bowel complaints for children.

P. F. Bowker, 1836

Take of prepared chalk 1 ounce, tincture of kino 1 ounce, Epsom salts 1 ounce, and water 1 pint; mix all well together, and shake well before using. Dose for a child 1 year old, 1 tablespoon morning, noon and night, and increase the dose as the symptoms may require.

Dr. A. A. Benezet, 1826

Infusion of tormentil root is beneficial in cases of weak bowels liable to frequent relaxations.

BOWELS INFLAMED

Take a tablespoon of St. John's wort oil nightly.

First take a tablespoon of olive oil and place hot water bag over the affected part. Change bag frequently, make up an infusion of elder flowers. Strain, add to this a little peppermint oil, stir well and give in frequent doses.

Steep 1 ounce of slippery elm bark bruised and sliced in 1 pint of boiling water for 2 hours in a closed vessel, then strain. Use freely as a drink.

Maidenhair fern made into strong tea is excellent where there is inward inflammation, and may be freely used, for it is perfectly harmless.

Take agrimony, cranesbill root 1 ounce, marshmallow root 1 ounce. Mix. Place ⅛ of the mixture in a vessel and pour on 1 pint boiling water. Allow to cool. Strain. Drink 1 wineglassful 3 times daily between meals.

45

Spermaceti is good in pain, and erosions of the intestines.

J. Monroe, 1824

Take 2 heaping teaspoons sweet gum bark and 2 heaping teaspoons of blackberry root; pour over 3 pints of boiling water, steep for 25 minutes or less and strain. When cold add mixture of powdered slippery elm mixed in cold water until smooth, then add 1 cup boiling water, stir well until mixture is not lumpy. Add to blackberry and sweetgum infusion. Keep in covered jar in refrigerator. Take 3 big swallows a day for either spastic or mucous colitis.

EXTERNAL APPLICATIONS

Bathe abdomen with solution of warm salt water. Massage with lard or olive oil.

Chop up a bagful red beets, warm a little and apply across abdomen.

Apply hops poultice to stomach and bowels.

Make a strong decoction of marshmallow leaves. Wet flannel with solution and apply as hot as can be tolerated.

BREASTS

TO DEVELOP

Drink freely of infusion made with goat's rue herb [*Galega officinalis*].

TO INCREASE MILK

The leaves or seeds of fennel boiled in barley water and drunk, are good to increase the milk when suckling child.

An infusion made with anise seeds taken first thing in the morning will increase both the quantity and digestibility of the milk.

Rosemary tea drunk in place of Oriental tea will increase the flow of milk of nursing mothers.

There is nothing that makes milk better than squaw weed for mothers of newborn babies as it does both in quantity as well as quality. Have had 13 babies born at my little hospital here and 2 had a shortage of milk so I just use squaw weed. It is fine and I can highly recommend it to all.

Mrs. H. H., 1916

TO DRY UP BREASTS

Apply freely an ointment made of bruised smartweed simmered in mutton tallow.

Take 4 ounces of strong tincture of camphor and add to it about 2 tablespoons of soft soap; shake well before using and apply to the breasts 3 or 4 times a day. Or, take 4 ounces of alcohol, ½ ounce gum camphor and castile soap; mix, and apply in the same way.

Sage tea given in cold infusion will within a few days cause the milk to leave the breast and prevent milk from forming where this is desirable in nursing mothers, as in cases of inflammation or gathering in the breasts.

Indians used the bruised leaves of tag alder as a poultice on breasts to stop milk.

SORE, SWELLED, HARD OR CAKED BREASTS

Apply hot pancakes made of sour milk, baking soda and wheat flour, large enough to cover affected parts. Keep them changed often so they will not be cold.

Bake large potatoes, put 2 or more in woolen stocking; crush them soft and apply to the breast as hot as can be borne; repeat constantly till relieved.

Miss E. Neill, 1890

Apply turnips roasted till soft, then mash and mix with a little oil of roses. Change this twice a day, keeping the breast very warm with flannel.

Take whiskey and soap—make a lather and apply to the breast.

Take soft soap and make a strong suds, and with a flannel cloth

well saturated with the suds, wash and rub the breasts downward
and with some degree of violence, once an hour; after which, each
time, bathe the breasts with polecat oil and camphor, and keep it
covered with a flannel. Pursue this course until a cure is effected.

C. Kinsley, 1876

Put on hot compresses for ½ hour, then rub with oil of spearmint
3 times daily until relieved.

Boil a quantity of chamomile and apply the hot fomentations.

Boil a handful of chamomile, and as much mallows in milk and water.
Foment with it between 2 flannels, as hot as can be borne, every 12
hours. It also dissolves any knot or swelling in any part where there
is no inflammation.

Take enough peach tree leaves to mix well with meal and water
to the consistency of a poultice. Apply hot but should not be used
where breasts have matter or pus.

Apply poultices of wild indigo to swelled female breasts.

SALVES FOR SORE BREASTS

Fry 1 pint of fresh hops in ½ cup of lard until the lard is a rich
brown, strain.

Take 1 pound of tobacco, 1 pound spikenard root, ½ pound comfrey
root, and boil them in 3 quarts of chamber lye till almost dry,
squeeze out the juice, add to it pitch and beeswax and simmer it
over a moderate heat to the consistency of salve. Apply it to the parts
affected.

Dr. L. Sperry, 1843

Take equal parts of plantain leaves and root, bittersweet bark, and
spignard root, boil out the strength, strain, and make it into an
ointment with hog's lard. This softens and relieves a caked breast
in a remarkable manner.

Take elder flowers and fry in lard, strain and bathe the breasts. It
will ease caked breasts at once.

Mrs. H. J. E., 1931

INFLAMED BREASTS

The best thing I have ever known to scatter the swelling and subdue the inflammation, if not gone too far, is the application of a mink skin—a fresh one is the best; but a dry one will do, by being softened in warm water. Apply it, or enough of it to cover the whole breast, with the flesh side next the breast, and continue to wear it there for some days, except when removed for the child to nurse, or to discharge the milk. It will sweat out the disease. It should be perfectly soft and pliant, and with the fur on. An ointment should also be applied occasionally, made by frying a little of the bark of bittersweet and jimson leaves in some lard.

If the swelling grows worse and is likely to gather, a poultice of powdered slippery elm moistened with warm lye water should be applied. When it has come to a head, so that you can see that matter has formed, it should be lanced; but it is always best to poultice and let it break itself. After it is open, continue the poultice, and wash the ulcer with the tincture of myrrh and aloes, occasionally injecting some into the opening. A decoction of wild indigo leaves and white oak bark is also very good as a wash. When the inflammation has been subdued by poulticing, heal with some good salve.

J. C. Gunn, M.D., 1862

SORE NIPPLES

When the infant stops nursing, apply clear molasses. This seldom fails to cure.

Apply a mixture with brandy and water. Wash off before baby nurses.

Always dry nipples after each nursing, and sprinkle with a little starch powder, or magnesia or grease with mutton tallow.

The oil of the nuts of the butternut tree make an excellent application.

Apply cocoa butter as a salve.

Apply an ointment made by simmering false bittersweet twigs or bark of root in mutton tallow.

Take 4 ounces of white wax, 1 ounce bayberry wax, 3 ounces spermaceti, 1 pint olive oil. Mix briskly over low fire, taking care to stir briskly until cool.

Make a strong tea of the bark of the root of bayberry, and wash nipples with it several times in a day.

Powdered comfrey root in a little water is excellent for sore nipples.

Apply jelly or mucilage made with quince seed. Soak seeds in a little hot water and strain off seeds before it becomes too thick.

Spread a plaster of fir balsam, and apply it to the breast after the child has nursed.

BRONCHITIS

Take honey, squeeze it out of the comb. Mix it with water and wet the mouth and lips frequently. A sure cure.

Dr. B. W. James, 1852

Take a teaspoon of lemon juice and olive oil the first thing in the morning.

Dissolve 1 cup of sugar in 1 cup of boiling water. Add 1 cup of olive oil and a pinch of ginger. Take wineglassful 3 times daily—one of the doses at bedtime.

Add a pinch of thyme herb to hot Oriental tea. Inhale the steam and drink the tea.

Ground ivy herb has been chiefly used in the treatment of chronic bronchitis, and its virtues in this affection are attested by medical evidence as well as by popular faith.

A. Stille, M.D., L.L.D., and J. M. Maisch, Phar. D., 1884

The syrup of coltsfoot herb is one of the best known remedies for chronic bronchitis. Make a strong decoction of the leaves, strain off the botanical and sweeten with honey. Take 1 or 2 tablespoons as needed.

Steep tablespoon of coltsfoot herb and tablespoon of plantain leaves in 1 cup of boiling water. Drink 2 or 3 cups a day.

Take of coltsfoot herb, elecampane root, extract of licorice, each

1 ounce; bloodroot ½ ounce; water ½ pint; good cider vinegar ½ pint; mix. Steep them near a fire, in a covered vessel, for 6 hours; strain, sweeten with molasses or honey, and flavor with essence of anise seed. Dose, from a teaspoon to a tablespoon 3 or 4 times a day. Good for chronic condition.

J. King, M.D., 1864

Take 1 ounce each of flaxseed, slippery elm, boneset herb and licorice. Boil in 1 quart of water—simmer until reduced to 1 pint. Add 1 pint vinegar and ½ pound sugar and simmer together. Take 1 tablespoon 3 or 4 times daily.

Take ½ ounce each of gentian root, prickly ash bark, skunk cabbage root. Steep in 2 quarts of best rye whiskey. Take teaspoon, drink slowly 5 or 6 times a day. A positive cure for bronchitis, even of long standing.

C. E. R., 1951

Take equal parts of horehound herb, hops, wild cherry bark, and licorice root. Make a strong decoction and add enough sugar to make a sirup and enough good whiskey to keep from souring. Take teaspoon as needed.

Take equal parts of the following: elecampane root, horehound herb, mullein leaves, bloodroot, black cohosh root, garden sage, musk root, golden seal root and comfrey root; add 2 parts skunk cabbage root. Mix thoroughly. Simmer 3 tablespoons in pint of water for 5 minutes. Allow to steep until cool. Strain. Take tablespoon as needed.

Mrs. J. J. C., 1948

Take ½ ounce each of horehound herb, Irish moss, whole flax seed, boneset and licorice root. Put in 2 quarts cold water then simmer until reduced to 1 quart. Take wineglassful 3 times a day. May be sweetened with honey if desired.

H. B. G., 1954

BURNS and SCALDS

Also see POULTICES.

For a dry burn, baking soda should be made into a paste with water.

For a scald or wet surface, the powdered soda (or borax will do as well) should be dusted on.

For mouth or throat scalded by hot liquid, gargle with borax water [dissolve an ounce of pulverized borax in a quart of soft water]. Give also slippery elm tea, and a little olive oil occasionally.

Stir baking soda in white of egg, and apply to the burn several times. It will draw fire and will not blister if applied quickly and not burned deeply.

L. M., 1931

Mix pulverized chalk and the whites of eggs to the consistency of cream. Apply to the burn. Relief from pain is instantaneous. Care should be taken by frequent application to prevent its congealing.

Plunge burn in cold water and add ice if available. Or apply cloths kept continually wet with coldest water possible.

Plunge the part scalded into cold water. Keep it wet with linen steeped in rectified spirits or common brandy.

Put ½ pound of broken camphor into a pint of good rum, keep it well corked in a bottle, apply it with a linen rag to the burn and the pain will be removed in a few minutes. Keep camphorated rum on hand for occasions needed. Label the bottle.

Put as much alum in a bottle of cold water as will dissolve, and keep it ready to apply immediately to a burn. Wet a cotton cloth in this solution, and lay it on the burn as soon as possible; when it becomes dry or warm, wet it again; it will ease the pain, and cure the burn in 24 hours, if applied before blisters are formed. The deepest burns have been cured in this way. For a small burn, where the skin is not broken, spirits of turpentine may be used.

Mrs. E. A. Howland, 1847

Lay a piece of smooth charcoal on the burn; the pain will subside immediately. Leave the charcoal on 1 hour and the wound will quickly heal.

Apply a poultice made with 2 parts corn meal, 1 part powdered charcoal and enough sweet milk to form a paste.

Apply a poultice made of oatmeal and cold water.

Vinegar applied every few minutes will keep burn from blistering.

Spread clarified honey upon a linen rag and apply it to the burn immediately, and it will relieve the pain instantly and heal the sore in a very short time.

Molasses and flour is the best thing for burns or scalds, no matter how severe. As soon as possible pour the molasses over the burn, then cover thickly with flour and wrap cloth around. The molasses keeps the flour moist and prevents it from pulling the little hairs in the skin, and both together keep the air out. If this simple remedy would be used before the doctor gets there with his linseed oil and cotton, many valuable lives would be saved.

If you burn your hand, put it in cold milk immediately and keep it there about 10 minutes, then dredge with flour or starch. Burns can be greatly relieved by covering with wet cloths dipped in a solution of alum—4 ounces to 1 quart water. Keep wet until healed. Powdered alum, fresh lard and white of egg mixed, is also very soothing.

Pie crust, without salt, is one of the best applications for a burn. Roll thin, and apply to the entire surface of the burn, and leave till it drops off. No inflammation or scar will remain but a second application may be necessary.

Make a poultice of grated raw potatoes, carrots, or turnips and bind to the burn. The poultice should be changed every hour until the burn heals.

Apply a poultice of pulped onion, well salted to the burn or scald and bandage securely. Pour salt water on the bandage until all swelling has subsided. Then apply a salve made with melted beeswax, olive oil and egg yolk thoroughly beaten together.

Mrs. A. B.

My mother does wonders with apple butter: A lady and man were in a bad gas explosion. The man ran to a doctor, he bandaged him up with an oil mixture while my mother spread on a thick coat of apple butter and kept adding it for a day or two. When the pain was gone and she was able to wash off the dried apple butter, her face never was scarred nor her hands or arms. But the man's face was red and a sight. His fingers are stiff to this day.

Old letter

Beat an apple with salad oil until it is a poultice, pretty soft; bind it on the part, and as it dries, lay on fresh. You must be sure to pare, core, and beat your apple well, for fear of breaking the skin of the burn. But if the skin be off, there is nothing in nature so sure to take out the fire.

Apply a poultice of fresh sauerkraut to the burn.

In case of burns, scalds, or frozen limbs, where the skin is off apply poultice of cracker meal and slippery elm powdered bark, made with raspberry leaf tea.

A poultice of tea leaves will afford almost immediate relief of minor burns.

The gel from the leaf blades of *Aloe vera* has long been used for burns. A 1937 report states the gel is also used for x-ray and radium burns.

The mashed fresh leaves of hens-and-chickens or houseleek, mixed with cream, gives quick relief for minor burns and scalds.

Take common pine tar, spread it on a cloth, put some oil on first, then apply immediately, and it will prevent blistering.

The bruised leaves of plaintain make a good application for burns and scalds.

Take the roots of white pond lilies, and roast them with hog's lard, to the consistency of a poultice, and bind it on the wound with a linen bandage. Leaves no scar.

Apply fresh mashed leaves of yellow dock to burns, scalds and blisters.

Apply the mashed fresh leaves of burdock.

The fresh juice of poke berries is very good for burns. The juice may be preserved by mixing with glycerine.

I suffered third degree burns over my arms, back, and hips, and after six weeks in the hospital, I was brought home and my husband steeped chestnut leaves, and after they were cool, placed the wet leaves over the burned area, covered with a cloth, and at intervals poured the tea over it. Our doctor was amazed at the rapid healing of the burns. This is twice I have experienced the value of chestnut leaves. The other time I was scalded by fruit jars blowing up, and we used nothing but the chestnut leaves. This is an old remedy.

Mrs. C. J. C.

Take the bark or berries of sumach, boil in milk and water, and make a poultice by stirring into it Indian meal. Apply this to the part affected, and repeat it as often as is necessary. This will effectually restore the muscles, and heal the sore, without leaving any scar. If this cannot be had, take basswood sprouts and scrape off the bark. Boil this in milk and water, and thicken it with Indian meal to the consistence of a poultice, and apply it to the part affected for 3 days, which will generally give relief.

J. Monroe, 1824

Take the bark of a sumach root, simmer it in cream, and anoint the part affected with this often.

For a very obstinate burn take the inner sole of an old shoe, burn it to ashes, sift the ashes, and sprinkle this on the sore. This will dry it up directly.

If you are on a farm and nothing else is available, use a poultice of cow manure when skin is not broken.

SALVES AND OILS USED

Take a tablespoon of lard, ½ teaspoon of turpentine, and a piece of resin as big as a walnut, and simmer them together till they are well incorporated; when cool, keep it in a box. In case of a burn, warm this so that you can spread it over a piece of linen, and apply it to the burn.

Mrs. E. A. Howland, 1847

Linseed or woodchuck oil are far ahead of most ointments for burns. Pour on the oil, put on cotton to keep out the air; then pour into the cotton more oil and wrap up.

Moisten burn with water, then apply peppermint oil.

The flowers and inner bark of common elder, simmered in cream or fresh butter, make a cooling ointment for scalds and burns.

The juice of beech tree which collects upon the inside of the bark in the month of June, mixed with an equal quantity of fresh butter or lard, makes an excellent salve for a burn.

St. John's wort oil applied freely, minimizes the pain of burns and scalds. The oil is made simply by steeping the flowering tops and leaves of St. John's wort herb (fresh or dried) in olive oil for a week or more. Leave the herb in the oil.

A bottle of carron oil should be kept in every house, ready for application on pieces of lint to scalds and burns. Carron oil consists of equal parts of linseed oil and lime water; it can be mixed at home, well shaken into a good size bottle tightly corked.

Take of fir balsam 1 ounce, sweet oil 2 ounces, mix, and apply with a feather, and then wet a cloth with it and lay it on the burn, keeping the cloth wet all the time.

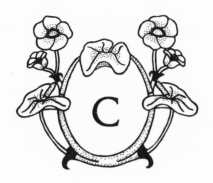

CARBUNCLES

Also see BOILS and POULTICES.

If the tumor should be likely to come to a head, or already have
done so, you should then touch it well with caustic potash. Burn
it with this at the points where it seems likely to open, and apply
poultices of slippery elm bark wet up with a strong decoction of indigo
leaves, or black willow bark, or of smartweed. Sprinkle a little
powdered lobelia on the poultice, before applying. Renew the poultices 2 or 3 times a day, applying the caustic well each time. When
openings appear, insert the caustic into them; and if you can get
the vegetable caustic, in powder, mix a little with double the quantity of powdered bloodroot, and sprinkle a little of it into the
openings and apply the poultice again. If there should be a tendency
to gangrene, or if the sore becomes large, angry, inflamed and offensive, wash with pyroligneous acid and tincture of myrrh, and poultice
with yeast, charcoal and slippery elm bark. The caustic should be applied at each dressing, until the tumor presents a healthy appearance.

J. C. Gunn, M.D., 1862

Puncture or open the tumor freely, and press out the contents, when
the slippery elm and ginger poultice should be applied, and renewed
once in 12 or 24 hours. At each renewal of the poultice the ulcer
must be washed with a tea of wild lettuce, xanthoxylon, or bayberry,
and then with a tea of cayenne, or tincture of myrrh, or both co-

joined. This last application is necessary to promote suppuration, that the head or core may be loosened and taken out.

Internally cayenne pepper, bitter tonic, diaphoretic powders and tincture of myrrh may be freely taken 4 or 5 times a day or oftener as the symptom may be, to guard against mortification. If mortification, however, should threaten or actually occur, a course of medicine must be immediately resorted to, and repeated as often as necessary until the bad symptoms abate; continuing also the other internal remedies. A poultice should likewise be made of sassafras bark or of smartweed bruised fine, boiled and thickened with corn meal, and applied to the part, or a yeast and charcoal poultice may be used instead of it, to prevent mortification. Fomentations of the smartweed bruised and boiled and applied hot, are also highly recommended to prevent mortification.

H. Howard, 1857

Take equal parts of sassafras root and slippery elm bark and make a strong decoction. Thicken with corn meal and apply as poultice.

Take a handful of fresh sheep sorrel leaves, wrap them in a cabbage leaf and roast in the oven. Apply as poultice as hot as can be borne.

Keep warm bread and milk poultice on until the core comes out, then keep covered with vaseline until healed.

CATARRH

MIXTURES FOR SNUFFS AND SMOKING

Take equal parts of pulverized sugar and finely ground borax. Sniff frequently.

Burn a piece of alum on the stove until it becomes a white powder, and use it as a snuff.

Eat raw onions daily; at the same time use a snuff made of white sugar, laundry starch, and burned alum, pulverized and mixed in equal quantities.

Take equal parts of black tea leaves with crushed cubeb berries and smoke in a pipe.

Take yellow dock root, split it and dry it in oven; bloodroot; scoke root, 4 ounces of each; cinnamon 1 ounce; cloves ½ ounce; pound them very fine, let the patient use it as snuff, 8 to 10 times a day. Every night smoke a pipeful of cinnamon with a little tobacco, and sweat the head with hemlock, brandy and camphor; pour a little camphorated spirits and brandy in the liquor to sweat.

Dr. L. Sperry, 1843

CHRONIC CATARRH

Take 1 ounce each of centaury herb, hoarhound herb, and marshmallow root. Place ⅓ of the mixture in 1 pint of water and bring to a boil. Simmer 15 minutes and strain. Dose, 1 wineglassful to a teacupful, according to the severity of the catarrh, 3 times daily.

CATARRH IN CHILDREN

When the disease first commences, the feet should be soaked in warm water, and the following remedy given: take pleurisy root, 1 ounce; ¼ ounce ginger, steep in 1 pint of boiling water, strain and sweeten. Give 1 tablespoon every 2 hours till relieved.

S. Pancoast, M.D., 1901

CATARRH IN LUNGS

Take 1 ounce of sulphur, 1 ounce of licorice-stick, 1 ounce of elecampane, pulverize them together, put in 2 tablespoons of honey; boil in 2 quarts of water to 1. Strain it off, and add gin enough to preserve it. For a dose, take 1 teaspoon 3 times a day, fasting.

CATARRH IN STOMACH

Steep 1 teaspoon of buckbean herb in 1 cup of boiling water. Strain when cool and drink 2 or 3 wineglassfuls daily as needed.

CATARRH IN BLADDER

Boil 1 ounce of rupturewort herb in 1 pint of water for 3 minutes. Strain and take a wineglassful 2 or 3 times daily.

Gipsy recipe

CHICKEN POX

No medicine is usually needed, except a tea made from pleurisy root, to make the child sweat. Milk diet is the best; avoidance of animal food; careful attention to the bowels; keep cool and avoid exposure to cold.

The finest combination on earth: 1 ounce boneset, 1 ounce scullcap, ¼ ounce goldenseal root, ¼ ounce powdered myrrh. Mix. Place the mixture in 2 pints cold water and cover. Bring very slowly to boil. Remove on boiling. Allow to cool. Strain. For the very young, 2 teaspoons every 2 hours; older children, 1 tablespoon every 2 hours. Sweeten with honey if necessary. Use a little witch hazel externally, for the irritable spots.

The bowels should be kept open by castor oil, and boneset tea administered to keep up the perspiration. If the stomach is full at the commencement of the disease an emetic of ipecac should be given. The diet low, as a matter of course.

Give patient freely of pennyroyal, sage, false saffron or catnip tea. If the bowels are confined give laxative. Sponge the surface of the body with saleratus water, and confine him to the house.

Bran tied up in a cheesecloth bag and patted on chicken pox sores will soothe and heal without scars. [Bag probably should be steeped in boiling water a minute or 2 before applying.]

CHILBLAINS

Also see FROSTBITE.

To relieve the intense itching of frosted feet, dissolve a lump of alum in a little water, and bathe the part with it, warming it before the fire. One or 2 applications is sure to give relief.

Wash the parts in strong alum water, applied as hot as can be borne.

Apply kerosene oil. Two applications will cure.

Application of turpentine often gives relief.

Paint the parts with a mixture of equal parts of iodine and ammonia.

Take teaspoon ammonia, strong; 6 ounces of rain water. Mix and bottle. Wet 2 or 3 folds of muslin with this mixture, bind on the inflamed part or parts for the night. Repeat this 2 nights. Gives great relief.

A solution of 30 grains of permanganate of potassia in an ounce of pure water, to be applied thoroughly with brush or swab, or in the form of a poultice.

Take 1 part muriatic acid, mingled with 7 parts water, with which the feet must be well rubbed for a night or 2 before going to bed, and perfect relief will be experienced. The application must of course be made before the skin breaks, and it will be found not only to allay the itching, but to prevent the further progress of the chilblains. Another good remedy is to dip the feet every night and morning in cold water, withdrawing them in a minute or 2, and drying them with a hard, coarse towel. If the feet are frosted, put them in a pail of brine.

Put the hands and feet once a week into hot water, in which 2 or 3 handfuls of common salt have been thrown.

Rub the part affected with brandy and salt, which hardens the feet at the same time that it removes the inflammation. Sometimes a third application cures the most obstinate chilblains.

In the evening, before retiring, take salt and vinegar made as hot as can be borne on the parts affected; bathe with a small cloth, and do so until cured.

Soak the feet in a weak solution of vinegar, then with vaseline or oil.

Bathe the feet often in cold water, and when this is done apply a turnip poultice.

Use 2 pints of the water in which parsnips have been boiled (no salt must have been added). Mix in the liquid 1 tablespoon of powdered alum. Stir well and bathe the hands or feet in the solution for 20 minutes. Then allow the solution to dry, without rinsing. Keep the solution for further use until the chilblains are quite gone.

Cook parsnips until tender and bind on the affected places; this simple application will often afford prompt relief.

Soak the feet well in water, then rub parts with sliced raw onion.

Slice raw potatoes, with the skins on, and sprinkle over them a little salt, and as soon as the liquid therefrom settles in the bottom of the dish, wash the chilblains; 1 application is all that is necessary.

Take the fat or tallow of a rabbit and anoint the part well once or twice a day, and especially at night on going to bed, and bathe it well by holding the part to the fire; and during the day, if the foot is the part affected, wear a bit of fresh rabbit's skin next to the affected part, with the flesh side next the foot. If there is much swelling of the affected part, with inflammation and soreness, poultice at night with rotten apples; or with slippery elm and ginger; or cover the part with warm glue. But in all ordinary cases, the use of the rabbit's fat and skin, will be sufficient. They will generally effect a permanent cure.

J. C. Gunn, M.D., 1862

Steep white oak leaves found on the trees during the winter season, and soak the feet several nights in succession.

Miss T. S. Shute, 1878

Take twigs of hemlock and pound them in lard until it turns green, then bind on parts affected.

Take common pine tar, spread it on a cloth, put some oil on first, then apply to frostbite. This is the best medicine ever used.

Rub hands or feet with juice of poke berries. I have known frozen inflamed feet to be cured in a few days with it. Bathe well and bandage with a cloth wet with the juice, cover with a dry cloth. Bandage night and morning. This is harmless even to a baby.

Mix together 1 ounce of turpentine and ⅜ ounce oil of sassafras. Apply the solution morning and evening.

Oil of spike or sassafras rubbed on twice a day will often effect a cure in a few days.

Wash parts with tincture of myrrh diluted in a little water.

CHILLS

In case of severe fatigue or chill from exposure, hot water is a harmless stimulant and will restore normal conditions very quickly.

Adults. Take a good shot of brandy or whiskey in a little hot water.

Take 1 teaspoon each of ginger, cream of tartar and sugar in a glass of very cold water.

Drink hot milk with a generous pinch of powdered ginger.

Take a pinch of cayenne pepper, a pinch of ginger, a tablespoon condensed milk, a teaspoon of brown sugar, and enough hot water to make a cupful. Drink up and you will find it sets you aglow inside at once.

Make an infusion with smartweed good and hot. Drink as hot as possible, go to bed and cover up.

CHOKING or SWALLOWING FOREIGN SUBSTANCE

Hold both hands high above head and gently tap between the shoulders.

When a child chokes on a bone or other object that it has tried to swallow, promptly turn the youngster upside down and hold it by the feet. In most cases the troublesome object will be quickly ejected.

Break a fresh egg in a glass and swallow whole egg. Or, take the white of several eggs and swallow. A little lemon juice will soften fish bones. Powdered bark of slippery elm infused in milk or water usually is effective for fish bone or other objects stuck in the esophagus.

Swallowing a large piece of orange pulp will force a fishbone or other substance into the stomach.

63

If you do not want a foreign object forced down, take a quick emetic. Warm grease of any kind generally will produce vomiting. Lard added to hot tea made of pennyroyal herb will produce vomiting.

Copper coin may be rendered harmless by a diet of bread and milk, giving nothing sour, as this would corrode the metal. Also give the raw white of an egg 3 times a day, and a dose of castor oil at night.

When a child has swallowed a button, or anything of that sort, the best way is to let him alone. Giving the child an emetic or a purgative will do him no good and may do a great deal of harm. If the thing swallowed has sharp or rough edges, give him plenty of potatoes and cheese to eat.

If your child swallows a pin or other sharp object and you are far from a physician, give at once a tablespoon of ground flaxseed or slippery elm bark mixed with just enough water to make a thick paste that will adhere to the foreign object, in a ½ hour give a teaspoonful of castor oil and beyond a doubt the pin will pass through the bowels wrapped in the pasty mixture. A noted physician gave me this remedy just before we came to western South Dakota,—50 miles from a doctor—to homestead and it saved my little girl's life.

Old letter

COLDS

Let a person fast for 2 days, providing he is not confined to bed, because by taking no carbon into the system by food, and by consuming the surplus which caused the disease, by respiration they soon carry off the disease by removing the cause. This will be found more effectual by taking copious draughts of water to continue fasting. By the time a person has fasted 1 day and night, he will experience a freedom from disease, and a clearness of mind, in a delightful contrast with mental stupor, and physical pain caused by colds.

Mrs. A. Matteson, 1894

For flu or colds, cut up a lemon like you would make lemonade. Put in a glass of cold water and drink unsweetened. Put more water over it and drink as long as strength is in it, then put up another one. Keep using as long as needed. A sure cure.

Mrs. F. J.

One lemon sweetened, pour on ½ pint boiling water. Drink just before going to bed. Be careful the next day.

Take a hot bath just before going to bed and drink a large cupful of hot lemonade or ginger tea. Put on heavy coverings until in a good perspiration; then gradually remove these until on the usual amount remains. Be careful about exposing yourself the next day.

Drinking this mixture hot before retiring, will often prevent a cold, after one has become thoroughly chilled: Slice up 1 lemon and remove seeds, add ½ cup sugar and 1 tablespoon ginger, and pour over 1 pint boiling water. Let it steep a little and settle. Drink it as hot as you can, and get into bed immediately.

Before retiring, drink a cup of hot water sweetened with brown sugar and some rum.

Sweeten Chinese black tea with honey, add a shot of brandy and a dash of nutmeg. Drink hot before retiring.

Make a tea with a mixture of black and green teas and add a little spearmint herb. Add the juice of 1 lemon. Drink 2 or 3 cups of this, piping hot on 2 nights before retiring.

Warm ½ pint of milk, and when on the point of boiling pour in ½ pint of molasses. Stir, and let it stand for 10 minutes, and then strain through muslin to separate the curds. Drink hot, and it will be found of great benefit.

Slice a few onions and boil them in a pint of new milk. Stir in a sprinkle of oatmeal and a very little salt. Boil until the onions are tender, then sup rapidly and go to bed.

Eating raw onions was believed to drive out a cold.

Upon the first intimation of a cold, take 6 drops of spirits of camphor upon a piece of sugar.

Make a decoction of white pine needles, sweeten with loaf sugar. Drink freely warm when going to bed and throughout the day.

Mayweed made into a strong tea, and used freely on going to bed, is an excellent remedy for a bad cold.

Make a strong tea made of either fresh or dried elder flowers, sweeten with honey and drink tea as hot as possible after the person is warm in bed; it produces a strong perspiration, and a slight cold or cough yields to it immediately, but the most stubborn requires 2 or 3 repetitions.

Taken in hot infusion with ginger upon going to bed, yarrow cannot be surpassed by any other herb for a common cold.

For colds or flu we use yarrow, peppermint, elder blossoms and ginger, simmered for 20 minutes. Drink a wineglassful every hour.

Mrs. R. L.

Peppermint is very hot in its nature, and may be used to advantage to promote perspiration and overpower the cold. Drink freely on going to bed.

Take a large draught of hot boneset tea on going to bed. A little peppermint may be added to prevent nausea.

Take 1 teaspoon boneset, 2 teaspoons dried mint, 1 teaspoon ginger, 1 teaspoon goldenseal root. Steep in boiling water 15 or 20 minutes. Strain and sweeten with honey. Take hot upon retiring. Also use a good laxative.

M. H.

Take a large handful of horsemint herb and boil in 1 quart of water until reduced to 1 pint. Strain and sweeten with honey. Drink glassful hot at bedtime.

Hot pennyroyal tea will often avert the unpleasant consequences of a sudden check of perspiration by a threatening cold.

Upon retiring, drink a hot decoction made of horehound herb, adding to each dose ½ teaspoon of cayenne pepper, with a tablespoon of good vinegar.

Every old lady in the country has more or less used dittany tea in colds. The tea is given frequently by infusing the leaves in hot water and drunk as warm as possible. It is a perfectly innocent plant.

J. C. Gunn, M.D., 1830

If you are attacked with chills, a pain in the breast, head, or back, bathe the feet in hot water just before going to bed and drink freely of a hot decoction made with wild ginger or snakeroot.

CHEST COLDS

A flannel rag, wrung out in boiling water and sprinkled with turpentine, laid on the chest, gives the greatest relief.

Use an onion poultice, which is made by heating the onions and putting them in a muslin bag and bruising them. Lay the bag upon the chest overnight. Care should be taken about getting in a draught when the poultice is removed in the morning.

Lay crushed flaxseed on a cloth, then macerate with a masher chopped garlic and onions on top of the flaxseed until it forms a moist paste. Lay the face downward on another thin piece of muslin and place on the chest and then place a piece of flannel or wool over that and a hot water bottle. The most stubborn congestion is relieved. Don't fail to likewise alkalize the body with a drink of some herb teas, such as senna with peppermint; cherry bark or nettle and by all means a quantity of citrus, lemon, grapefruit or orange.

Rub chest and throat with skunk's oil. It penetrates and relieves congestion.

Put hops or catnip in a bag and steep in hot water for few minutes. Apply as poultice on lungs and throat as hot as can be tolerated. Produces local and general perspiration.

HEAD COLDS

Dissolve a tablespoon of borax in a pint of water; let it stand until it becomes tepid; sniff some up the nostrils 2 or 3 times during the day, or use the dry, powdered borax like snuff, taking a pinch as often as required. At night have a handkerchief saturated with spirits of camphor, place it near the nostrils so as to inhale the fumes while sleeping.

Rub the dried flowers of sneezeweed to a powder then sniff it up the nose. It will cause sneezing and clear the nasal passages. Repeat if necessary.

Pour a cupful of boiling water over a teaspoon of thyme and add 2 drops of oil of peppermint. Sip slowly.

As soon as you feel that you have a cold in the head, put a teaspoon of sugar in a goblet, and on it put 6 drops of camphor, stir it and fill the glass ½ full of water; stir, till the sugar is dissolved, then take a dessertspoonful every 20 minutes.

A colored janitor in the neighborhood who is very old, yet very capable in his work, originated from about 50 miles out of Memphis. His relatives and ancestors all lived to be over 100 years and are on the same plantation where they were once slaves. He told me that for generations whenever one had a head cold or grippe, the dried herb of rabbit-tobacco was smoked in a corn cob pipe.

E. O., 1965

Symptoms of cold in the head are quickly relieved by spraying, with witch hazel, both the throat and nasal passages.

If the nose is stopped up so that it is almost impossible to breathe, smoke crushed cubeb berries in a pipe. Emit the smoke through the nose.

Put pine tar on hot coals and breathe the fumes.

Letter, 1931

HEAD COLDS IN CHILDREN AND INFANTS

Cleanse nostrils with tepid warm water, then rub camphorated oil over the whole surface of the nose, being careful not to go into the eyes of infant. Repeat when necessary.

The oil of sweet marjoram, diluted with water, and applied to the nose of infants, when they are so stopped that they cannot suck, generally gives relief.

When baby's head is all stopped up with a cold, grease the bottoms of his feet, palms and nose thoroughly with pure lard, and see how quickly relief will follow.

COLIC

A few tablespoons of hot water [not scalding] will often allay a severe attack in children. Adults take a glassful. Hot water may be sweetened with molasses or brown sugar.

For adults. Sweeten a glassful of hot milk with a little sugar; drink while hot. Repeat in 15 minutes if not relieved. Or drink a glassful of hot milk in which 1 teaspoon of ground nutmeg has been added.

Make a tea with 1 teaspoon of ground ginger to a pint of boiling water. Steep 3 or 4 minutes, then strain. Dose, 1 to 2 teaspoons for children to be repeated in ½ hour if not relieved. Adults may take wineglassful at a time.

Dissolve a teaspoon of salt in a glass of warm water; give in teaspoon doses every 5 minutes for children. Tablespoonful doses for adults.

Make a tea of dried orange peels [not dyed]. Strain and drink infusion while warm. Children or adults.

Aniseed, fennel seed, caraway seed, are among the best and most popular colic remedies for infants, as well as children and adults, used in domestic practice. The infusion is made with a teaspoon of any one of the above seeds, steeped in boiling water. Strain off seeds in 3 or 4 minutes and sweeten a little if desired. Give infants 1 to 3 tablespoons; children more according to age; adults wineglassful or teacupful. Infusion should be given warm.

Give a scruple of powdered aniseed in child's food.

Give child 5 to 6 drops oil of aniseed on a lump of sugar.

Put 5 drops oil of aniseed and 2 drops of oil of peppermint on ½ lump of sugar, rubbing it in a mortar, with 1 drachm magnesia, to a fine powder. A small quantity of this may be given in a little water at any time, and always with benefit.

A drop of essence of peppermint in 6 or 7 teaspoons of hot water will give relief. If the stools are green and the child is very restless, give warm chamomile tea. An injection of a few spoonfuls of hot water into the rectum with a little asafoetida is an effective remedy.

An infusion made with peppermint leaves or spearmint herb makes a soothing home remedy for infants, children and adults troubled with colic or gas. Use 1 teaspoon of mint to 1 cupful of boiling water. Strain before infusion becomes cold. Give infants 1 or 2 tablespoons of the warm infusion; children several swallows; adults 1 cupful. Sweeten if desired.

Warm catnip tea is an old favorite and a sort of panacea for children and infants with colds or colic.

If the baby seems to suffer from colic and acidity of the stomach and bowels, a ¼ teaspoon of powdered slippery elm bark, thoroughly mixed with sugar and added to the milk with which the baby is fed, may give relief. Slippery elm is harmless.

Mrs. E. B. Duffey, 1882

An infusion made with balm acts like a charm. Place 2 teaspoons in a teacup filled with boiling water. When cool, strain, and give hourly, 1 to 2 teaspoons to children over seven.

A tea made of flowering dogwood blossoms is recommended by many for colic in children.

The leaves of peony made into a weak tea, are good for infants when troubled with wind in the stomach.

Wild black cherries dried and pounded fine are a good remedy for colic.

One drop of camphor in a teaspoon of water will often relieve colic in children.

Steep 1 tablespoon of snakeroot or wild ginger in a cup of warm water for several hours. Strain and give to children in teaspoonful doses as needed.

An infusion made with 1 teaspoon of ginseng root steeped in 1 cupful of boiling water for 5 minutes. Strain. Give to infants 2 or 3 teaspoons while tea is warm. Give children more according to age; adults may take cupful at a time.

Make a tea of calamus root, sweeten and give a teaspoon to the child whenever there are signs of trouble coming on.

Take 2 ounces sweet flag, 1 ounce marshmallow roots, ½ ounce powdered ginger. Mix. Steep 1 teaspoon in a cup of boiling water. Strain. Drink ½ cupful or full cup while warm. Children less according to age.

Take equal parts of ginseng root and white root, ½ as much calamus or angelica seed, dry them, pound very fine, and mix together. A teaspoon is a dose for a grown person; for children, less according to their age. Repeat the dose once in ½ hour if required. This rarely if ever fails.

Steep a teaspoon of yarrow leaves and flowers in 1 cup of boiling water. Strain before it cools completely and drink a wineglassful while still warm.

A spirituous infusion of the berries or the bark of the prickly ash, is made use of in Virginia in violent colic. The fresh juice expressed from the root, affords certain relief in colic, and what is called dry bellyache.

Take ½ drachm of powdered rhubarb, and toast it a little before the fire. Then add a little powdered ginger to it, and mix it for 1 dose for adults, to be repeated as occasion requires.

EXTERNAL APPLICATIONS

A towel folded several times and dipped in hot water and quickly wrung and applied over the seat of the pain will generally afford prompt relief.

Habitual colic. Wear a thin soft flannel on the part.

When the baby is troubled with colic, rub the abdomen well with warm sweet oil, and it will cause relief almost at once.

Apply outwardly a bag of hot oats, or steep the legs in hot water a ¼ of an hour.

For a person afflicted with the bilious colic, take the bran of corn meal, make it into a pudding, sprinkle mustard over it, and apply it, as hot as can be borne, to the bowels. Drink hot peppermint water.

Fomentations of hops; stramonium leaves and hops; lobelia herb and hops; or wormwood and boneset herb, etc. may be used, and applied warm over the whole stomach and bowels.

CONSTIPATION

Begin with 1 newly laid hen's egg [raw], add it to 3 times its bulk of cold water; let it be beaten for 30 minutes to the finest consistence. Take it in the morning on an empty stomach, and once or twice in the course of the day afterwards; continue for 8 to 10 days, increasing the quantity from 1 to 3 at a time, if the stomach will relish them; and they will gradually and pleasantly remove costiveness and strengthen the system.

A cup of hot water, as hot as one can drink before breakfast.

A tablespoon of olive oil 3 times a day for weak or very old people. It may be used as an enema when it cannot be tolerated.

A pinch of salt in a glass of water taken before breakfast.

Take glauber's salts 1 ounce, manna ½ ounce, dissolve them in a little boiling water for 1 dose, to be taken as often as occasion requires.

Stew figs slowly in olive oil until plump and tender; add a little honey and lemon juice and allow to boil until thick.

Steep 1 ounce senna leaves in 1 pint boiling water until strength is extracted. Place a layer of figs in an earthen dish and pour over them the strained senna tea. Place the dish in a moderate oven and allow to remain until the liquid has been absorbed by the fruit. Keep in a closed jar. Take 1 fig as a dose before retiring.

A similar recipe: One pound of best figs, 1 ounce of senna, the senna to be pounded and made fine as possible; the figs to be chopped fine; to be well incorporated together; a very little molasses to be added, to make it of a right consistency. This is a very gentle cathartic. To be taken in pieces as large as a chestnut.

Take in powdered form: 2 ounces senna, 1 ounce jalap, ½ ounce mayapple root, ¼ ounce cloves, ¼ ounce bicarbonate of soda. Mix well. Take 1 teaspoon in a cup of boiling water and sweeten once a day. Children less according to age.

Take of jalap 1 pound, alex senna 2 pounds, peppermint plant 1 pound. Let these articles be pulverized and sifted, then mix them together. Dose a teaspoon or 1 drachm. It should be put in a teacup with a lump of loaf sugar and a gill of boiling water added. When cool, give it to the fasting patient. This forms the best general purge known. It is useful in all diseases known where physic is required; in serious and bilious diseases it is invaluable.

Take of the infusion of senna, 2 ounces; syrup of buckthorn, 1 ounce; mix them together for 1 dose, which may be taken in the morning fasting, 3 times a week, and it is a safe and sure purge; it may be taken in all cases where purging is proper.

Take buckthorn berries [*Rhamnus cathartica*], and boil them in water, until all the strength is out. Strain off, and press the berries hard. Then add 1 pint of molasses to the same quantity of juice, and simmer it as long as any scum rises, which must be taken off as fast as it rises. When it stops rising, stir it well and put it up for use. If the weather is warm, add gin or brandy sufficient to keep it from souring. A large teaspoon is a dose for an adult. If it causes any griping, it may be easily remedied by steeping a little caraway seed [*Carum carvi*], with it, which will prevent its having that effect. It is very safe, but powerful, if taken in large doses, as are also the dry berries. From 3 to 7 berries are a smart dose for a grown person. They lose their strength by age, especially if exposed to the air.

P. F. Bowker, 1836

Take 2 teaspoons of flaxseed and stir into a cup of cold water and let it stand ½ hour. Drink seed and all.

The leaves and blossoms of the peach tree purge the bowels freely, and without the least griping, when taken as a strong tea, in doses of a teaspoon every hour: they also act as a mild purgative when taken as a syrup, prepared by boiling slowly their juice, with an equal quantity of honey, sugar or molasses, and given to children in doses of a tablespoon, and to grown persons in doses of a wine, or stem-glassful.

J. C. Gunn, M.D., 1830

The leaves of thoroughwort, powdered fine, and mixed with molasses, is a gentle purge, and good to create an appetite.

The juice of the common elder berries, when ripe, is good for those troubled with costiveness, being physicking and entirely harmless.

The butternut [*Juglans cinerea*] bark pills, are a valuable purge, very easy and safe, to all persons under disease. These pills may be prepared by boiling a kettle of the bark of the butternut tree in water, until you gain the substance of the bark, then strain the liquor and boil it down; when it becomes thick as syrup, take care not to burn it, but simmer it to a substance like hard wax; then put it by in a cup or galley pot, and make it into pills as they are wanted, for if the pills are made up, they will run together and dissolve in a little time. This purge is preferable to any that I know, in a weak and debilitated state of the bowels. It may be taken in as small quantities as you please, for if they do not purge immediately, they act the better as a stimulus and tonic to the system, and will produce a good habit by repeating them every night, and this may be done for a month together. This differs from all other purges that I know of in this—that your doses may be less and less, but other physic must be more and more, or it will not purge. Other purges generally leave the body in a worse habit, but this in a better. Its general ease and safety, and its answering in almost every disease, so that I venture to say the trial of it will never be wrong, make it a far preferable medicine to salts or any other purge, where repeated applications are wanted. I advise to begin with 1 or 2 pills a night going to bed, which may be swallowed in a little stewed fruit or rye mush, and the doses may be increased a little every night till they purge; then take less and less till the patient is quite well.

P. Smith, 1812

Butternut extract 1 ounce; rhubarb root ½ ounce; aloes ¼ ounce; cayenne ⅛ ounce; lobelia seed ⅛ ounce. Mix and make into pills. Take 1 every hour until an action is produced.

Mayapple root is an emetic and cathartic: if 2 teaspoons of the powdered root be taken at once, it will operate both as an emetic and cathartic; but if the same quantity be divided into 6 or 8 portions, and 1 of them be taken every 15 minutes, it operates as a cathartic only. The extract, made into pills, has the same effect.

Man-root is a moderate laxative: it opens the system in general, relieves pains of the stomach and sides, and corrects the digestive powers; it is commonly prepared in syrups, teas and bitters.

Boil 1 ounce of the bark of alder tree in a pint of water for 5 minutes. Dose, a wineglassful at night.

At night place 5 or 6 cloves in a teacup, and ½ fill it with boiling water. On arising in the morning drink the cold clove water.

An infusion of 1 ounce of cascara bark to a pint of boiling water; infuse for 1 hour and strain. Dose, 1 teaspoon, morning and evening or according to needs.

A decoction made of the bark of young white ash acts as a gentle aperient or cathartick.

Dr. D. Rogers, 1824

Other botanicals used for their carthartic properties: bark of root of Indian physic [*Gillenia trifoliata*]; Culver's physic root [*Leptandra virginica*]; Bowman's root [*Apocynum cannabinum*]; purge-root [*Euphorbia corollata*] and many others.

CONSTIPATION IN INFANTS AND CHILDREN

Rub the abdomen with a firm gentle motion from left to right with olive oil.

One-half teaspoon olive oil, ½ teaspoon orange juice, 3 times a day after feeding.

Simmer a few prunes in enough water to cover them for ½ hour, with tablespoon senna leaves. Remove the prunes and allow to dry. Let child eat prunes when needed.

Manna is a gentle purgative, so mild in its operation that it may be given with safety to children, persons of very weak habits, and in pregnancy.

The blow [flowers] of common elder makes a physicking tea, that is good for children.

P. F. Bowker, 1836

CONVULSIONS

Put the child, as quickly as possible, up to his neck in a warm bath about blood heat; keep it so by careful addition of hot water. Put a napkin wrung out of cold water around his head, and let him remain 10 to 15 minutes. Then take him out and wrap in a warm blanket, and usually he will be all right. Diet is the great prevention in most cases. If the convulsions are accompanied by frothing at the mouth with bloody tinge, it is usually epilepsy, which is seldom cured or outgrown, and little can be done except to keep the patient from hurting himself.

Mrs. M. W. Ellsworth, 1897

Convulsion fits sometimes follow the feverish restlessness produced by these causes; in which case a hot bath should be administered without delay, and the lower parts of the body rubbed, the bath being as hot as it can be without scalding the tender skin.

Miss E. Neill, 1890

Convulsions may be sometimes cut short by turning the patient on the left side.

Fits can be instantly cured by throwing a spoonful of fine salt as far back into the mouth of the patient as possible, just as the fit comes on.

To cure this distressing form of malady, take 2 pennyworth of camphor, and infuse it in 1 pint of brandy. Let it stand 48 hours, and then it is fit for use. When the attack comes on, take 1 teaspoon in a wineglass of water.

Drink a decoction made with equal parts of bittersweet root and scullcap herb. Boil a tablespoon of the mixture for 3 or 4 minutes in 1 pint of water. Strain when cool. Take a wineglassful 3 times a day or as needed.

Take 2 ounces of Peruvian bark and 1 ounce of steel dust, tincture in 1 pint of good wine. Take a wineglass 3 times per day. As the paroxysms decrease lessen the quantity to 1 glass per day.

Dr. B. W. James, 1852

A tea made of the roots of convulsion weed [*Monotropa uniflora*] dried and taken in a powder, is good for convulsion fits.

Pulverize equal quantities of dried sage and white sugar and take some every morning before breakfast for several weeks.

A tea made of the blueberry root [*Caulophyllum thalictroides*], when it comes to be known and proved, will probably be esteemed as the best antispasmodic in the compass of medicine. That is, it will prevent and do away spasms of every description in a safe, and superior manner. By spasms I mean involuntary contractions—such as cramp, hiccup, cholic, cholera, morbus, epilepsy, hysterics, and I suppose every other species of fits, even ague.

P. Smith, 1812

COUGHS

For tight, hoarse cough, where phlegm is not raised, or with difficulty, take hot water often, as hot as can be sipped. This will be found to give immediate and permanent relief.

A pinch of salt will stop coughing at night.

A pinch of a mixture of salt and sugar, taken now and then, will help to loosen an obstinate cough. Use 1 part salt to 2 parts sugar.

A teaspoon of hot honey taken every ¼ hour will break up the worst cold in one day. It will also relieve severe spasms of asthma.

Children with slight cold, cough or throat trouble: give teaspoon every hour strained honey with ¼ lemon juice.

To 2 ounces glycerin add juice of 1 lemon and 4 ounces of pure honey. Give in doses of 1 or 2 teaspoons as often as needed.

Mrs. E. N., 1949

To 1 cup molasses add 2 tablespoons dark brown sugar and ½ lemon, cut fine. Boil over slow fire until it begins to thicken, then remove and add 1 tablespoon glycerin and vinegar enough to give a sharp taste. Dose: 1 teaspoon whenever cough is troublesome.

Take 1 cup of strained honey, ½ cup olive oil and the juice of 1 lemon. Cook 5 minutes, then beat thoroughly for 3 minutes, so that ingredients will mix. Take 1 teaspoon every 2 hours.

To 1 pint of boiling water, add pinch of cayenne, slice of lemon, 3 tablespoons honey, 1 ounce cut slippery elm bark. Allow to stand ½ hour, and strain. Take frequently in small doses.

Heat 1 cup of milk nearly to a boiling point. Add a piece of stick cinnamon and a tablespoon of butter, drink the milk while warm.

Take a lump of butter, some vinegar, cinnamon and enough sugar to sweeten; mix with some water and boil it down to make a thin syrup.

Take 1 ounce of butter, 1 ounce of honey, and a sprig of rosemary, in ½ pint of milk, and drink going to bed. Molasses may be used instead of honey.

Take 3 yolks of hen's eggs, 3 teaspoons of honey and 1 of pine tar; beat them well together, add to them 1 gill of wine. Take a teaspoon 3 times a day before eating.

One pint best vinegar, break into it an egg and leave in shell and all, overnight. In the morning it will all be eaten except the white skin which must be taken out. Then add 1 pound loaf sugar, and for an adult, take a tablespoon 3 times a day. This is a most excellent remedy for a cough in any stage.

An onion cough syrup is made of 6 large onions cooked in 1 quart vinegar until soft. Strain and squeeze out all the juice, add 3 pounds sugar, and when cold add 2 ounces tincture of lobelia. Very good for sore throat, and especially croup.

Take 18 ounces of good onions, and after removing the rind make several incisions, but not too deep. Boil together with 14 ounces of moist sugar and 3 ounces of honey in 35 ounces of water, for ¾ hour; strain and bottle. Give 1 tablespoon slightly warmed immediately on attack, and then, according to needs, 5 to 8 teaspoons daily.

Take a large beet, make a deep hole in the center, fill with sugar or honey and bake until done. Eat some every time you feel like coughing.

Mrs. R. S., 1951

Put coarse sugar between sliced turnips, give syrup in teaspoon doses.

Put 1 pound fresh ripe blackberries into a pan with 2 tablespoons of water and cook very gently till all the juice is drawn out. Strain through a muslin bag and then leave to get quite cold. To every tablespoon of juice mix 2 tablespoons of honey and one dessertspoonful of glycerine. Keep well corked and sealed. Dose a dessertspoonful 4 times a day.

Equal parts of good vinegar and water, and to a teacupful of this mixture add 1 teaspoon of the best African cayenne, and sweeten with honey or sugar. Dose, 1 tablespoon, which will allay the cough instantly. A dose taken at bedtime will generally enable the patient to rest well all night; if, however, the cough becomes troublesome at any time before morning, another spoonful will allay it.

Take ¼ pint white vinegar, 2 ounces honey, ¼ ounce licorice extract, 1 lemon. Place the vinegar and licorice extract in a basin. Put into a very hot oven and stir until licorice dissolves. Add honey, and when cooling add the juice of the lemon. Instead of putting into the oven, the vinegar and licorice can be boiled in an enamelled pan over a very gentle heat. Dose, take 1 tablespoon whenever the cough is troublesome. It is an excellent thing for children with weak chests and is a preventive as well as a remedy.

To 1 cup of boiling water, add 1 or 1½ jiggers of whiskey and 1 tablespoon butter. Drink as warm as possible.

Take equal parts of whiskey and pepper sauce and mix with honey to make a syrup. A teaspoon every time cough is troublesome.

One pint of 100 proof whiskey, 4 ounces glycerine, 4 lemons. Put lemons in moderate hot oven so juice may be extracted easily. To the above ingredients add 1 pint of pure honey. Boil all ingredients together 20 minutes. Bottle.

Mrs. C. P., 1948

For hard, unyielding coughs: one gill of molasses, 1 gill new rum, 2 teaspoons pulverized licorice, and a piece of alum as large as a walnut.

Take equal parts of olive oil, honey and Jamaica rum; mix well together. For an adult, 1 tablespoon 3 times a day; for a child 3 months old, from 10 to 15 drops—increase the dose according to age of child. If the cough is very severe, take the preparation when inclined to cough, always shaking well before using.

Make a syrup of sugar and brandy and add a little sweet oil. Dose, 1 teaspoon when needed. Shake bottle each time before using.

Boil 2 ounces of flaxseed in 1 quart of water; strain and add 2 ounces of rock candy, ½ pint of honey, juice of 3 lemons; mix, and let all boil; let cool and bottle. Dose, 1 cupful before bed, ½ cupful before meals. The hotter you drink it the better.

Take 1 teaspoon flaxseed; 1 ounce licorice; ¼ pound raisins. Put ingredients into 2 quarts of water, and boil it down with a slow fire to ½ the quantity, then add ¼ pound rock candy pounded fine and add 1 tablespoon lemon juice. Dose, ½ pint on going to bed, and take a little when cough is troublesome. This recipe generally cures the worst colds in 2 or 3 days. It is a sovereign balsamic cordial for the lungs.

Take 1 quart thick flaxseed tea, 1 pint of honey, ½ pint of vinegar, 2 teaspoonfuls saltpeter. Boil all together in an enameled container, until it becomes a thick syrup; keep stirring while boiling with fresh pine stick. Dose, 1 tablespoon 3 or 4 times a day.

Soak ½ cup of whole flaxseed in ½ a pint of boiling water. In another dish soak a cupful of broken bits of slippery elm also in ½ a pint of boiling water. Let both soak for 2 hours or more, then strain both through a fine cloth into a porcelain lined dish and set on to boil with 2 pounds of granulated sugar. After boiling hard for 10 minutes add the juice of 2 lemons and boil until it turns to candy. Test by dropping a few drops into cold water.

One handful of hops; pour boiling water on it; simmer with 1 tablespoon of flaxseed, for 15 minutes. Strain. Add 1 teacup of sugar, and a little slippery elm bark. Boil up again; add the juice of a large lemon. Pour into a bowl, taking 1 tablespoonful at a time.

A tablespoonful each of flaxseed and Irish moss simmered together for 15 minutes in 1 pint of water and flavored with liquorice and honey, and then strained, is soothing and helpful last thing at night.

Make a tea of equal portions of flaxseed and coughwort, boil them well together, strain the liquor, and use it with honey. Use it many times in the day and night.

Boil a handful of coughwort leaves in a quart of water till reduced to a pint, sweeten with rock candy, and acidulate with a slice of lemon. A wineglassful to be taken 3 or 4 times daily.

Take of horehound a small handful, and about as much coughwort, 2 tablespoons of sage, and 1 of false saffron, well simmered together. Strain off botanicals, add ½ pint of molasses, and simmer it again for 3 hours, with moderate fire, and while it is hot, add 1 gill of the best Holland gin. Dose, 3 times a day. Commence with a tablespoon, and increase to ½ wineglassful. This is a safe remedy and may be relied on for a cough of any kind, except the whooping cough.

Make a strong infusion of ½ ounce horehound herb in ½ pint boiling water. Add this to ½ pint whiskey, with ¼ pint glycerin, ¼ pound rock candy.

Take ½ pound of horehound herb, 3 tablespoons flaxseed and 3 table-spoons ginger. Boil all in 3 quarts of water, then strain and add 1 pound granulated sugar. Boil slowly, stirring often, until reduced to 1 quart of syrup. Take 1 or 2 teaspoons 5 times a day.

Make an infusion of horehound herb; sweeten with honey, and make hot with cayenne. Add teaspoon of vinegar.

Take ½ pound horehound, 1 pod of red pepper, 4 tablespoons ginger. Boil together in 3 quarts of water until all the strength is removed. Add 1 tablespoon of good pine tar and 1 pound brown sugar. Boil slowly and stir often until reduced to 1 quart of syrup. Dose 1 or 2 teaspoons 4 or 6 times a day. Very good.

Mrs. D. D., 1931

Simmer together 1 ounce mullein leaves and ½ ounce horehound herb in a quart of soft water till strength is extracted (add more water if necessary); strain and add 1 pint molasses. Dose, 1 table-spoon 3 times a day.

Take 1 ounce of horehound herb, 2 ounces black cohosh root and 2 ounces skunk cabbage root; boil in 3 pints of water down to 1 quart. Strain, and add ½ ounce saltpeter and 2 pounds sugar or honey. Dose, 1 teaspoon 3 or 4 times a day.

The root of skunk cabbage is excellent for a cough, by being grated on honey and swallowed.

Peach leaves and twigs are useful in a bad cough; steep down to a strong tea with about ½ the quantity of skunk cabbage, add the same quantity of good molasses as there is of the tea, take ½ wineglass 3 or 4 times a day.

Take 3 tablespoons of ground comfrey root; 3 tablespoons ground spikenard, and 1 teaspoon skunk cabbage root. Steep in 1 pint boiling water. When cool, strain and add the juice of 2 lemons and ½ cup strained honey. Take 1 teaspoon every 2 hours and it will stop the most severe cough.

One ounce essence hemlock [*Tsuga canadensis*], 2 ounces castor oil, 1 pint molasses, 1 teaspoon camphor; mix essence, oil and camphor together, and shake thoroughly; then add to the molasses. Dose: teaspoon from 4 to 6 times a day. Though simple, it has accom-plished wonderful results.

Take the inside bark of a pine tree, steep and sweeten with strained honey and boil down to a syrup. Take tablespoon as needed.

Put about 3 quarts fresh picked white pine needles in earthenware kettle, cover with water and let soak over night. In the morning put over the fire, and when it comes to a boil push back where it will simmer slowly several hours. Strain and add 1 pound sugar and boil to a syrup, then strain again and add ½ pint gin, and bottle. One teaspoon every hour till relieved. Has cured many obstinate coughs, especially those left by grippe.

Put 5¢ worth of pine pitch into a pint of water. Let it simmer until the water is well impregnated with the flavor. Dip out the gum which remains undissolved and add honey enough to sweeten and make a thick syrup. Strain this and bottle. Dose, a teaspoon 4 or 5 times a day, according to the severity of the cough. It will afford speedy relief.

Take 4 parts each of wild cherry bark, and life everlasting herb, 2 parts each of spikenard root and horehound herb, 1 part each of elecampane root, and licorice root. Steep 1 ounce of the mixture in 1 pint of boiling water. Strain, add rock candy or honey to make syrup. Take in teaspoon doses.

Mrs. A. J., 1916

Take a small handful of wild cherry bark and boil in about 1 quart of water until the strength is out. Strain off the bark then add an equal amount of honey to the strained decoction. Boil until a good syrup consistency and take a teaspoon every 3 or 4 hours through the day.

Mrs. I. L. D., 1931

Take 2 ounces of balm of gilead buds, the freshest you can procure, and boil them very slowly in a quart of water. Let it simmer down to 1 pint, then strain it, and then add 1 pound of honey in comb, with the juice of 3 lemons. Let them all boil together until the wax in the honey is dissolved. This has been known to cure a cough of long standing.

Take of balm of gilead buds 2 ounces, balsam of fir 1 ounce, good gin, or whiskey, 1 pint; mix. Let them stand 10 or 12 days, frequently shaking, and strain. Also take 6 ounces of sunflower seeds, bruise them, and slowly boil them in 3 pints of water down to ½ pint, then strain and add above gin tincture. This may be sweetened, if desired, with honey or sugar. Dose, a tablespoon 4 or 5 times a day.

Make a strong tea of boneset herb; to a quart of the tea add a quart of molasses; boil it down to a thick syrup: when cool, bottle it for use, and keep it in a cool place.

Take 1 ounce of boneset herb, 1 ounce slippery elm, 1 ounce stick licorice, and 1 ounce of flaxseed; simmer together in 1 quart water until the strength is entirely extracted; strain carefully, add 1 pint best molasses and ½ pound loaf sugar; simmer them all well together, and when cold, bottle tight. Take tablespoon as needed.

Simmer in 3 quarts of water, 1 pint of barley, 4 ounces of elecampane root, and 1 pound of turnips; boil these and after it is strained, simmer it down to 1 pint; add 1 pound loaf sugar or honey, and ½ pint of brandy. Take a tablespoon 3 times a day for a hectic cough.

Take ½ pint honey, 3 tablespoons elecampane root powdered, 3 tablespoons ginger, 1 pint of vinegar. Put all in a jug, and make a paste of flour or chop-stuff, and shut the jug close up with this paste; and then, when you put your bread in the oven, put this jug in also, and leave it in the oven until you take the bread out; then it is ready for use. Dose, 1 teaspoon 2 or 3 times a day, and as you can stand it.

Take a handful of hops, put it into 3 pints of hot water; let it boil ½ hour, or until the strength is out. Strain and add 1½ cups of molasses, and 1 cup of white sugar. Boil down slowly in enameled kettle to about 1 quart. Then bottle up, and it is ready for use. Drink a little when you cough.

Boil about 1 ounce of dried mullein leaves in 1 pint of water till reduced about ½. Strain off the herb and add enough loaf sugar to make a syrup. Dose for an adult, a tablespoon after each meal and before retiring.

Boil ½ ounce yellow dock root in ½ pint of water to make a strong decoction. Strain when cool, add enough honey or brown sugar to make a syrup. Dose, 1 tablespoon 3 times a day. Most wonderful cough syrup according to old source.

Gum myrrh will cure a recent cough by adding molasses and hot water; it should be drunk warm.

Keep a piece of ginger root in the mouth and chew it like tobacco; swallowing the juice is very good for cough.

A strong tea made of the berries or bark of scarlet sumach is excellent in cough, either the common or whooping cough; add about ⅓ good molasses.

Coughs of long standing. Make a strong decoction of ground ivy herb, strain when cool; sweeten and thicken with honey or brown sugar.

The roots of marshmallow boiled in wine, or honey and water, are good for coughs, hoarseness, shortness of breath and wheezings.

A decoction of feverfew herb, with sugar and honey put thereto, may be used with success to help a cough and stuffing of the chest, by colds.

Make a decoction of pyrola herb. Strain off the herb and add brown sugar or honey to make syrup. The leaves of pyrola are also chewed for colds.

Honey and wild Indian turnip make a good remedy for colds, coughs, etc. Grate the turnip root and mix with honey. Take a teaspoon for a dose. [Not for children.]

Make a strong decoction of the round roots of sedge grass [*Cyperus rotundus* or *C. esculentus*], strain and add to honey or molasses to make a sirup.

Kentucky recipe

DRY COUGH

Make a thickish tea with slippery elm bark or a strong decoction of sage leaves. Sweeten if desired.

Take ½ ounce powdered gum arabic; dissolve it in hot water, and squeeze in the juice of a lemon, add ½ ounce of licorice juice, 2 drachms of paregoric, 1 drachm of syrup of squills. Cork all in a bottle and shake well. Take 1 teaspoonful when the cough is troublesome.

Take licorice, and boil it in spring water, with some maidenhair fern and figs, and use it for constant drink. It is good for diseases of the breast and lungs.

For a dry irritating cough, smoke in a common clean pipe equal quantities of ground coffee and pine sawdust. Swallow all the smoke you can. Gives instant relief.

CROUP

As soon as the wheezing is heard apply the coldest water to the neck and chest. Pound up some ice in a napkin and feed the child a little at a time with a spoon. Keep the cold compress on the throat and chest, and if persisted in for a short time relief will be almost certain to follow. At any rate, even if a physician is sent for, use these precautions, and 9 times out of 10 the disease will be checked. The chief danger is in delay; there is not an instant to lose.

Mrs. Owens' New Cook Book, 1897

A strip of flannel or a napkin folded lengthwise and dipped in hot water and wrung out, then applied around the neck of a child that has the croup will usually bring relief in 10 minutes.

A warm bath will frequently relieve the worst paroxysm: or bathing the feet in hot water and rubbing with heated flannels. Small doses of hive syrup may be used as an emetic.

Miss M. C. Cooke, 1889

At the very first sign of wheezing, active measures should be pursued. Let no time be lost in giving an emetic—immerse the feet in warm water and put a poultice of yellow snuff, mixed with goose oil, or sweet oil, upon the stomach. Apply several thicknesses of flannel, wet in hot water, over the throat, as hot as can be borne, and change as often as it cools. Put onion poultices on the feet, after soaking them a little time; lose no time in sending for a physician.

Mrs. E. A. Howland, 1847

The best remedy which can be given to a child attacked with croup is an emetic. A wineglassful of lamp oil or goose oil will often answer this purpose, where no better medicine can be obtained. The best emetic which can be given to a child in the croup is a heaping tea-spoon of powdered alum, mixed with molasses or honey. This should be given every 10 minutes, until it pukes freely. The alum operates on the salivary glands and makes them pour out the saliva or spittle in great quantities.

J. C. Gunn, M.D., 1862

Croup can be cured in 1 minute and the remedy is simply alum and sugar. The way to give it is to shave or grate in small particles about a teaspoonful of alum; then mix it with about twice its quantity of sugar, to make it palatable, and administer it as quickly as possible. Almost instantaneous relief will follow.

Miss T. S. Shute, 1878

Boil pig's feet in water, without salt, and let it stand overnight; in the morning skim off the fat which will be formed in a cake on top, put this in a tin pan, boil until all the water is evaporated; bottle and keep for use. Give a teaspoon every 15 minutes on the appearance of the first symptoms, and apply freely to chest and throat, rubbing well.

Warm a teaspoon with a little lard in it or goose grease; thicken with sugar, and give it to the child; it may produce vomiting which is always desirable, thus breaking up the membrane that is forming. Apply lard or goose grease to the throat and chest, with raw cotton or flannel. Care should be taken, removing only a small piece at a time of these extra wraps to prevent taking cold.

Dip a piece of fat meat in kerosene oil and bind it to baby's throat.

Letter, 1931

A teaspoon of flour of sulphur to 1 glass of water given every hour has wonderful effects.

Take equal parts of alcohol and water, and give in small quantities.

Slice onions thin, putting them in a stewpan with just enough water to keep from burning, and stir in a little corn meal. The onions may be used alone. Apply to throat and lungs, as warm as can be borne.

Get 3 red onions and slice them up fine and fry them in 1 pint of lard until a light brown, then give child a teaspoon every 15 minutes till it vomits—it will never have croup again.

Take and cut onions in thin slices, between and over them put brown sugar and let it dissolve. A teaspoon of the syrup will give immediate relief.

Steep several hours sliced onions or garlic in a jar of honey. Give teaspoon every 15 minutes until relieved.

One teaspoon of beet juice given every 5 minutes will help in cases of croup.

Administer a small teaspoon of powdered bloodroot in molasses; if this does not afford speedy relief, repeat the dose in ½ hour.

Take 1 handful of fresh chamomile, 1 handful of false saffron blows, either fresh or dry, and 3 ounces of fresh butter, simmer them together over a moderate fire, till the flowers become crisped. Give a teaspoon of this oil every 20 minutes, till it affords relief. This dose is for a child 1 or 2 years old.

DEBILITY

Also see FEMALE WEAKNESS, TONICS and BITTERS.

For weakness and general debility of the whole system: Take of lovage root ½ pound, 4 ounces of burdock root, and ½ pound of comfrey root to 4 quarts of water, and let it boil moderately for the space of 2 hours, strain it off and then continue to boil it down to 1 quart, add ½ pint of the best Holland gin, and 1 pound of honey, or loaf sugar will do if honey cannot be procured; put it into a bottle, and cork it tight for 8 and 40 hours, when it will be fit for use. Dose: a tablespoon 3 times a day before eating. This syrup has been known to perform a great many cures after every other remedy had failed.

P. F. Bowker, 1836

For all sorts of inward weakness, pains in the stomach or breast. Take 4 pounds of red clover flowers, 20 pounds fir boughs and 1 pound of spikenard. Mix these with 10 gallons of cider, and put them into a still. Draw off 3 gallons and drink ½ gill at night and morning.

Sarsaparilla [*Aralia nudicaulis*] sweetens the blood and juices; it is good in debilities, and should be taken in strong decoction.

J. Monroe, 1824

An infusion of the flowers, or light decoction of the leaves of betony, or a saturated infusion in rectified spirits, is good in laxity and debility of the viscera, and disorders arising from thence.

87

Sweet fern is very purifying and strengthening. A tea of any part is good in all cases of debility, indigestion, relax or dysentery.

Indians gather the leaves of sweet fern in September and drink an infusion of it the year round.

For weakness of either sex, make a sirup of Solomon's seal root, and life-of-man root, and sweeten it with honey, and drink freely and frequently.

Large Solomon's seal roots [Convallaria multiflora] are mild, yet very healing and strengthening; commonly prepared in syrups, and administered in cases of consumption and general debility. Small Solomon's seal [Convallaria racemosa] roots have properties similar to large Solomon's seal.

Dr. D. Rogers, 1824

Decoctions of goldenrod herb are excellent in weakness and debility. There are 2 kinds: the largest of these is the strongest.

DEBILITY OF THE AGED

The milk of a woman is called better than any other kind for medical uses. When this is taken in cases of extreme debility, it should be sucked from the breast of a middle aged woman, of good habits, who lives temperately, and uses moderate exercise. The patient should suck about four hours after the woman has taken her meals. Milk drunk immediately after it is taken from the cow, is likewise of great benefit in consumptions, and cases of debility, if it agrees with the patient: if not, it may be churned.

J. Monroe, 1824

An egg, taken in spirit every morning in cases of extreme debility, has often performed an effectual cure.

Take 1 pint of good cider vinegar, drop into it a few pieces of soft iron; nails, or pieces of nail rod is the best; let it stand and the vinegar will burn black. You can use this with or without wine. If you have wine take 1 part iron-mixture and 2 parts of any kind of wine, mix. This remedy is good for female irregularities, general debility of old people, for coughs that sirups have no effect on, and should be used for a month or so at a time. Dose for adults 10 to 15 drops; for children, less.

The most distressing weakness, with which delicate constitutions are so often afflicted, may be better cured by simply substituting the following beverage for the usual drink of beer, ale, etc. at meal times, during a few days or weeks, according to the degree of weakness, than the most costly and complicated medicines—Boil as much pearl or Scotch barley, in pure water, as will make 3 pints; then, straining it off, and having in the meantime dissolved an ounce of gum Arabic in a little water, mix them, and just boil the whole up together. The barley water need not be thick, as the gum will give it sufficient consistence. When used, take it milk warm; the good effect will generally be soon manifest, and a complete cure certainly follow.

The Family Receipt Book, about 1800

Elderly people of both sexes will find the following a very useful preparation, viz., buchu leaves, spleenwort leaves, balmony herb, of each 1 ounce; ginger ½ ounce. Put down in 3 pints of water, boil gently to 1 quart, strain, and take a wineglassful 2 or 3 times a day, sweeten if desired. This is a very valuable preparation for the aged and infirm, as well as for those troubled with general debility; or where it may be stated, that no particular part of the system is diseased, but the languid, depressed, debilitated state demands a remedy.

Mrs. A. Matteson, 1894

White poplar bark is a good remedy for old people and for those who have been brought low by disease. It is the most renovating medicine that can be employed; it is excellent for loss of appetite, and combined with buchu leaves and juniper berries makes one of the very best compounds as a general restorative. Take 2 ounces each of the above mentioned articles, bruise the berries and boil gently for 2 hours in 3 pints of water; strain and sweeten, and take a wineglassful 3 times per day.

DIARRHEA

Also see BOWEL COMPLAINTS and DYSENTERY.

INFANTS AND CHILDREN

In case of violent pain, apply cloths wrung out of hot water to the belly. If the belly is hard, and sore on being touched, grease it well with any kind of oil or lard. The frequent use of the warm bath will be of immense service.

For babies use either the seed or root of burdock mixed with yeast and bandage on the navel. Do not remove until mucus, blood, etc. stops. It takes 3 to 7 days.

Mrs. A. B.

One or 2 teaspoons of Chinese tea at intervals often will stop diarrhea in infants. Tea may be sweetened.

Give carrot soup diet for infants.

Give babies a little carob or St. John's bread flour in warm water or boiled milk every 4 hours.

OLDER CHILDREN AND ADULTS

Give older children raw apple or bananas.

Let the child drink slowly a teacupful of boiled milk as hot as possible.

For children troubled with a relapse. Take ½ cup of new milk, and add to this 2 teaspoons of good brandy, and scald it. After it cools, feed the child with it freely, and continue this for several days. It will effect a cure.

Give child or adult 1 or 2 teaspoons of thick cream every hour.

Parched corn is an excellent remedy for dysentery, diarrhea and bowel complaints in children. Parch some corn, then grind fine in a coffee grinder. Boil in sweetened and salted milk and feed the patient. It is a palatable and healthful food generally relished by children. Let them eat as much of it as they please.

A remedy more adapted to children, is to parch ½ pint of rice until it is perfectly brown, then boil it down as is usually done, and eat it slowly, and it will stop very bad diarrhea in a few hours.

Scorched flour in boiled milk or scorched flour and sugar eaten dry.

For children, mix a little flour in boiled milk together and give them a teaspoon every hour.

Burn an ordinary-sized cork till it is completely charred; then reduce to a fine powder, mix with it an equal quantity of loaf-sugar, a teaspoon of brandy, a little grated nutmeg, a teaspoon of essence of peppermint, and a tablespoon or 2 of water, and give it to children in teaspoon doses. It is innocent, and may be given frequently, and in larger quantities. Good in diarrhea, cholera morbus, summer complaint of children, and bilious colic.

For children or adults drink a tea made from dried orange peels [not dyed] and use as a common drink for 24 to 36 hours. Tea may be sweetened with loaf sugar.

Take a glass of hot lemonade every hour or ½ hour.

To a wineglass of warm water add 1 tablespoon of vinegar, and 1 teaspoon fine salt. Take this at 1 dose, and if it does not afford relief in ½ hour, repeat the dose. The second dose is almost sure to give entire relief. This is said also to give relief in case of bilious colic.

Mix together 3 teaspoons salt, 4 teaspoons black pepper and ½ cup each of cider vinegar and warm water. Take 1 tablespoon every 30 minutes, or more in severe cases. For adults only.

For children with diarrhea or dysentery: Take the roots of cat-tail flags, wash them clean, and boil them in milk. Sweeten it with loaf sugar, and feed them with it every day.

A few leaves of sessame plant steeped in cold water makes a clear mucilage which has been highly extolled for bowel complaints of children, to be given as a common drink.

Boil in 1 quart of water 1 ounce of dewberry root. Boil down to ½ pint. Take ½ wineglassful 2 or 3 times a day in severe cases. Reduce doses as discharge diminishes.

Boil 1 ounce of alum root in 1½ pints of water for 20 minutes or until the liquid is reduced to 1 pint. Dose, a small wineglassful twice daily for children over 5 years old. Decoction may be sweetened.

The center leaves of mullein steeped in milk, and sweetened with sugar, are an excellent remedy for diarrhea or dysentery, especially for children.

Boil 2 or 3 stalks of garden mint in milk. When liquid is cold take a wineglassful 3 times daily.

Boil comfrey root or slippery elm bark in milk. The botanicals add a soothing quality.

The inner bark of white pine boiled in milk often is effective.

The oil extracted from mutton suet, cures a diarrhea in a short time. The dose for an adult, is 1 tablespoonful.

To a ½ pint fresh, new milk add stick or ground cinnamon enough to flavor, and white sugar to taste; bring to boiling point, and take either warm or cold. Excellent for diarrhea in adults or children. A few drops or a teaspoon of brandy may be added, if the case demands.

Put into a bottle 3 ounces allspice upon which pour 1 pint best French brandy; sweeten with sugar. Dose: a wineglassful every hour for 3 hours for adults. For children, dilute, and give 1 tablespoon each hour. This remedy has been known to cure violent cases of diarrhea.

J. Marquart, 1867

Drink a tea made with allspice; follow with a tea made of slippery elm bark.

Beat up an egg, grate in ½ a nutmeg and sweeten to taste. Repeat 2 or 3 times during the day.

Make a poultice of all kinds of spices, heat whisky and wet the poultice, apply to the stomach and bowels.

Take 2 handfuls of the root of blackberry plant to 3 pints of milk and boil down to 1 quart. Dose, 1 cupful every 2 or 3 hours.

The root of blackberry must be boiled a long time in order to get out the strength—after the strength is out boil in a little milk and sweeten it, and let the patient drink at liberty.

P. E. Sanborn, 1836

Drink either blackberry wine or brandy in small doses or eat the canned blackberries when fresh fruit is not available.

Mrs. E. B. B., 1958

Give a child blackberry jam.

To 1 quart blackberry juice add 1 pound sugar, 1 tablespoon each of cloves, allspice, cinnamon, and nutmeg. Boil all together 15 minutes, then add a wineglass of whiskey, brandy or rum. Bottle while hot, cork tight and seal. This is almost a specific in diarrhea. One dose, which is a wineglassful for an adult—½ that quantity for a child—will often cure diarrhea. It can be taken 3 or 4 times a day, if the case be severe.

Boil 1 ounce of rhubarb root for 5 minutes in 1 pint of water. A small dose will cure. A large one is a safe aperient.

Take 1 heaping teaspoon of golden seal root, 1 heaping teaspoon rhubarb root and 1 heaping teaspoon baking soda. Dissolve in ¾ cup of water and let come to a boil. Dose for a child with a very bad diarrhea 1 teaspoon every ½ hour until the movements are the color of the medicine—usually 6 or 8 doses, then 1 teaspoon 3 times a day for 2 or 3 days.

Take equal parts of crane's-bill root and golden seal roots. Boil table-spoon of this mixture in 1 pint of water for 10 or 15 minutes. Strain and drink 1 cup or more as needed for adults.

Take equal parts of powdered white or red oak bark and slippery elm in cold water. Drink freely.

Dried leaves of shepherd's purse, taken in red wine, form an efficacious remedy in diarrheas and where astringents are indicated.

Chew the buds of common ragweed and swallow the juice.

An infusion made from boneset herb will cure diarrhea. One half cup will usually stop the symptoms, but it is best to take several cups more over the following days to build yourself up.

C. H., 1964

The root of water avens is a popular remedy in diarrhea. A decoction is made and taken with sugar and milk in the same manner as coffee.

Barton recommended the leaves of sweetfern for diarrhea, loose bowels and the summer complaint of children, or cholera infantum, in the form of a weak decoction; but it is used in Pennsylvania and Virginia for many other diseases, such as all children's bowel complaints (where it forms a grateful drink for them) in rachitis, in debility, in fevers as a diluent tonic.

C. S. Rafinesque, 1828

An infusion of the leaves and flowers of *Spiraea tomentosa* was in common use in colonial New England as a domestic remedy in diarrhea and other complaints where astringents are required.

CHRONIC DIARRHEA

Drink freely of boiled milk to which 1 teaspoon of powdered gum arabic or slippery elm bark has been added.

Take hardwood ashes, 3 tablespoons; cider vinegar 3 tablespoons; hot water enough to cover; stir it well, then let it settle. Give 1 teaspoon of the liquid every little while.

The following is very good for chronic looseness. Bistort root 3 ounces; water 1 quart. Boil 20 minutes, then add 1 ounce of cloves, cranesbill root and wild mint, of each ½ ounce; catechu 2 drams. Boil 10 minutes longer, strain, add loaf sugar 1 pound. Dose, 3 tablespoons 3 or 4 times a day.

DIET DURING DIARRHEA

Tea without milk, and very little sugar; mutton and chicken broths, or beef tea, thickened with a little flour or arrowroot; boiled rice, tapioca, sago; rice water or toast water to drink. If the attack is severe or of long continuance, the patient must be kept in bed. The feet must be kept warm, and the covering to suit the feeling of the patient.

*The Modern Home Cook Book
and Family Physician,* about 1880

DYSENTERY

Eggs beaten up slightly with or without sugar, tend to lessen the inflammation of the stomach and intestines, and by forming a temporary coating on these organs, enables nature to resume her healthful sway over the body. Two or at most 3 eggs a day would be sufficient in ordinary cases; and since the egg is not merely a medicine but food as well, the lighter the diet other than this, and the quieter the patient keeps, the more certain and rapid is the recovery.

Take the yolks of 3 eggs, 2 ounces of loaf sugar, 1 gill of brandy, and 1 nutmeg grated; the whole to be well mixed. A grown person should take 1 teaspoon every 2 or 3 hours; children less, according to age.

Give a teaspoon of prepared chalk in a little cold water 3 times a day.

Burn a piece of white bread into almost charcoal. Put it in a glass of ice water, or as cold water as you can get. Drink nothing but this water all that day. It will stop in an hour's time and will stop vomiting too. Do not take anything to move the bowels.

Letter, 1931

A broth made of the meat of sheep is a very wholesome diet in dysenteries.

Many are in the habit of giving castor oil in dysentery, but I prefer olive oil. It seems to sheathe the intestines, and defend them from acrimonious humors. After the mucilaginous teas a tablespoonful of olive oil may be given in a little milk, or other article every morning. It usually acts as an aperient or laxative.

W. Beach, M.D., 1833

Good vinegar and as much salt as it will dissolve; add 1 tablespoon to 4 of hot water, take as fast as it can be, and as warm as can be. This dose to be continued every 2 hours till it acts as physic.

Take salt and vinegar sweetened with loaf sugar.

Two ounces of fine salt in 1 pint French brandy, and taken a teaspoon at a time 2 or 3 times a day, will soon give relief. This is also good for rheumatism, dyspepsia, and indigestion.

Into ½ glass of port wine stir a teaspoon of starch, sweeten with loaf sugar; grate ½ nutmeg in it; drink 3 or 4 times a day.

Take 2 wineglasses each, sweet oil, good molasses, and West Indian rum, and simmer them well together over a fire till they become the thickness of honey, so that the oil will not separate from the rest; while on the fire, keep it well stirred, and when taken off, continue the same till it is cold. A grown person should take a tablespoon once an hour, till he finds the disease abating, then once in 2 hours, or as the judgment may suggest. Children to take in like manner, in proportion to their ages.

One pound of wild cherry bark, 1 pound sweet gum bark, 2 pounds brier root, 1 gallon of rum and enough loaf sugar to sweeten.

Take of cherry-rum and brandy, each ½ pint, ½ pound of loaf sugar, 2 ounces of essence of peppermint. Dose, 1 spoonful 2 or 3 times a day.

Ripe blackberries 2 quarts; loaf sugar 1 pint; cayenne ½ ounce; cinnamon ½ ounce; cloves ½ ounce; allspice ½ ounce. Boil all together for a short time; when cold strain and add a pint of brandy. Dose, from a tablespoon to a wineglassful, according to the age of the patient. It is sometimes well to produce perspiration by covering the patient warmly in bed and giving warm drinks of flaxseed, balm, sage or catnip tea. If this does not produce perspiration, give 2 grains of ipecac every 3 hours.

The berries of elder bush in all forms, fresh, dried or cooked are good in dysentery.

Take a quantity of ripe sweet elder berries, press out the juice, simmer it over a slow fire, add some brown sugar, and let it set till it becomes a thin syrup. Then add ⅓ the quantity of brandy and cork it up tight in a bottle. It is then fit for use. If a grown person, take a wineglassful for a dose. If a child, ½ the quantity will be sufficient. It may be taken 3 or 4 times a day. This medicine has proved good in many cases where all other remedies have failed.

Take 1 teaspoon of pulverized maple charcoal, mix it well with a tablespoon of molasses, then add 2 tablespoons of fourth-proof West India rum, and ½ a glass of sweet oil; mix the composition well together, and for an adult let it all be taken at 2 doses. If it does not stop the complaint (as it seldom fails), take a smart dose of castor oil, and after it has operated, repeat the above composition. This is decidedly the most effectual remedy that we have ever used in inveterate cases of dysentery, or any complaint of the bowels.

For dysentery in its worst form. Take the bark from the root of a spruce, and scrape it up towards the body of the tree. Dry this and pound it fine, sift it through a fine sieve, mix a teaspoon of this with ½ glass of warm water, and drink it. If this does not answer, repeat the dose again in 2 hours, which will generally be sufficient. After this, make a strong tea from the inner bark of witch hazel, sweeten it with loaf sugar, and add a little milk. Drink of this freely.

Take 3 ounces of white pine bark, after the ross is off, and 3 pints of water; simmer it down to 1 quart, strain it off, and then add to it ½ pint of West India molasses, and ½ pint of West India rum. If the patient be a grown person, take the whole; for a child, half. This remedy, though simple, seldom fails.

Mix the inner bark of hemlock tree, with boiling water, sweeten a very little, and use it freely. It will be sure not to have any bad effect.

The Indians cure the most obstinate dysentery with a decoction made of the bark of sassafras roots.

Take 1 tablespoon rhubarb pulverized; 1 tablespoon peppermint pulverized; 1 tablespoon saleratus; ½ pint boiling water: when cold, add a wineglass of brandy, and sweeten with loaf sugar. Dose, ½ wineglass once in 2 or 3 hours, till the disease is checked.

Take best turkey rhubarb root, saleratus, peppermint plant, cinnamon pulverized, of each 2 scruples, take tablespoon every hour till the passages are changed.

Rhubarb root 1 ounce, English saffron 2 drams, and 1 nutmeg, bruise the whole well in a mortar. Put them in a pint of brandy of the first quality, cork the mixture, stand it in the sun or before the fire 48 hours, shaking it occasionally. It will then be fit for use. Dose, teaspoon to be taken 3 times a day. It rarely fails.

Rhubarb 4 ounces, black cohosh root 2 ounces, wild cherry bark 2 ounces, crane's bill root 2 ounces. Mix, and pour on the articles, 2 pints of brandy and 2 pints of water. Let mixture stand 5 or 6 days, frequently stirring, and then strain. Add 4 pints of water to the dregs, boil down to 2 pints, strain, and add to the strained liquor the previous tincture, and sweeten with loaf sugar. Dose, tablespoon every 1 or 2 hours.

In mild cases, use the pulverized rhubarb root burnt to ashes in an iron vessel, stirring it until it turns to a black color, or is well burnt. Give a ½ teaspoon, or less, 3 or 4 times a day, swallowing it with a little water; will often check the disease in a few hours.

Mucilaginous drinks are beneficial, such as an infusion of slippery elm, bene plant, marshmallows, etc. They may be given alternately as the stomach will bear. Slippery elm is decidedly the best article. It possesses very gentle and anti-phlogistic properties. A teaspoon of the pulverized bark may be stirred into a tumbler of cold water, and the whole or part given as the patient is able to take it. Three or 4 teaspoons may be given through the course of the day.

Take powdered guaiacum 5 drachms; mucilage of gum arabic 3 ounces; simple syrup 3 ounces; water 8 ounces. Mix. Dose, ½ wineglassful every 4 hours.

Tormentil is a powerful astringent, and a sure and efficacious medicine in diarrheas, dysenteries, and hemorrhages; but must be used with caution, lest the flux be stopped too soon.

J. Monroe, 1824

Make an infusion by steeping the herb Canada fleabane in hot water. For dysentery take a cupful every hour or 2 until relieved.

Roast the seeds of common burdock in a closed vessel. Pulverize like coffee. Take 1 level teaspoon in a cup of boiling water, sweeten with honey if desired. Drink 1 cup upon rising, 1 cup an hour before lunch, and 1 cup upon retiring. In less than a week the mucus, the blood, the terrific painful stool becomes normal. In very severe cases the root of burdock is washed, cut, boiled and drunk as above. Do not use too much of the root.

Mrs. A. B.

An infusion made with horsetail grass is good for bloody flux.

Mouse-ear is one of the best articles now known for the dysentery. To prepare it for use, boil a small handful of the herb in a pint of milk and water, sweeten it with a very little loaf sugar, and use it freely for drink. It is perfectly harmless, and is most certain to cure the disorder.

Steep a tablespoon of the herb and flowers of toadflax in 1 cup of boiling water for a few minutes; sweeten. Take wineglassful several times a day.

The bark of white oak was reckoned the best remedy which had as yet been found against the dysentery. It is reduced to a powder, and then taken: some people assured me, that in cases where nothing would help, this remedy had given a certain and speedy relief.

P. Kalm, 1772

Take equal parts red oak bark, wild cherry bark and blackberry roots and make a strong decoction. Drink ½ to 1 wineglassful at a time as needed.

Spotted spurge [*Euphorbia maculata*] is used for bloody flux and dysentery in Old Indian Territory—always with good results. We take a handful of weed and put it in ½ gallon of water and make a tea of it. Dose, ½ cupful 3 times a day. This remedy was given my mother by a Choctaw Indian and I have seen same used many times with great benefits.

This is an old soldier's remedy for cholera infantum and diarrhea in old and young. Pull up the weed [spotted spurge], wash and cut it up about 1 inch long and boil in milk, pressing off and on, as it boils, with a tablespoon to get all the milky substance out of the weed. I have seen children given up by doctors, get well with just a very few doses. This old soldier said, when he was in the army, a number of soldiers died of cholera that were treated by the doctors, while he didn't lose a case; all those who followed his advice, taking this spotted spurge got well. It is also good dried for use in winter.

Old letter

Spotted spurge or spreading spurge has been used widely among negroes of the southeastern states. Related varieties of spurge [*Euphorbia hirta* and *E. Glyptosperma*] used for bloody flux by natives of the West Indies.

CHRONIC DYSENTERY

A decoction made of black birch inner bark is good for all bowel complaints, and excellent in case of dysentery.

Take 1 ounce each of bayberry bark, wild cherry bark, black birch bark and bitter almonds. Boil ingredients in 1½ quart of water until reduced to 1 quart. Sweeten with loaf sugar, and add a gill of brandy. From ½ to 1 wineglassful may be taken 3 or 4 times a day on an empty stomach.

Boiling water poured over equal parts of sumac berries and red raspberry leaves makes a useful drink in chronic dysentery.

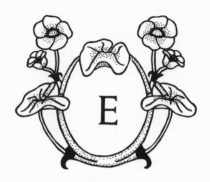

EARS

EARACHE

Apply a warm poultice or rub in back of the ear with warm oil. In case of a discharge, syringe the ear with warm water.

Insert cotton plugs dipped in a warm mixture of glycerine and witch hazel, or glycerine and rosewater. It may also be relieved by rubbing around back of the ear with equal parts of turpentine and lard.

Take a tablespoon of fine salt, and tie it up in a little bag, heat it quite hot, and lay it on the ear, shifting it several times; and it will afford speedy relief.

Take 2 quarts of warm water as warm as the child can stand it; add 5 teaspoons of table salt. Flow gently into the ear from a syringe or pitcher. In severe cases do this every 2 hours till the child goes to sleep.

Mrs. U. J. A., 1944

Drop a little fresh warm milk into the ear.

Soak the feet in warm water, roast an onion, and put the heart of it into the ear as warm as can be borne. Heat a brick and wrap it up, and apply it to the side of the head. When the feet are taken from the water, bind roasted onions on them. Lard or sweet oil dropped in the ear as warm as can be borne, is also good.

C. Kinsley, 1876

Take a small piece of cotton wool; make a depression in the center and fill with black pepper; gather into a ball and tie up; dip it in sweet oil and insert it into the ear. Almost instant relief will be experienced. Juice from a roasted lemon is good. A piece of salt pork cut in a strip and inserted in the ear will give relief.

Steep a clove of garlic in warm olive oil for a few minutes and put into the ear, rolled up in muslin or fine linen. When the garlic has accomplished its object, and is removed from the ear, it should be replaced with cotton to prevent the patient taking cold.

Warm fresh leaves of rue on the stove and roll them in cotton and put in the ear.

C. F. S., 1914

Take a green stick off an ash tree, put it in the fire, catch the juice as it bubbles and put it in the young 'uns ear. Hot coffee in the ear is good too.

Dissolve asafoetida in warm water; while warm drop several drops in the ear, then cork the ear with cotton.

Mix ½ ounce oil of sassafras with 1 ounce olive oil and 1 dram camphor. Warm this liniment and pour a small quantity on a pledget of cotton, and bind over the ear. If pain continues drop small quantity of above mixture in the ear.

Roast a piece of lean mutton, squeeze out the juice and drop it into the ear as hot as it can be borne.

REMOVING FOREIGN SUBSTANCE FROM EAR

Take a horse hair about 6 inches long, and double it so as to make a loop at one end. Introduce this loop as deeply as possible into the auditory canal, and twist it gently around. After 1 or 2 turns, according to the originator of the plan, the foreign body is drawn out with the loop. The method is ingenious, and at all events causes little pain, and can do no harm.

Hard substances, such as peas, beads, etc. occasionally get lodged in the passage of the external ear. If the substance be within sight, and can be grasped readily with a small pair of forceps, that will be the best way to extract it; but force must not, on any account, be used. The safest plan is to inject lukewarm water rather forcibly into the ear by means of a syringe, one that will hold at least 2 ounces. This will be found rarely to fail, the water passing beyond the substance, and being there confined by the membrane, called the tympanum, forces the former outwards. Should the substance have swelled, or the ear become swollen, a little sweet oil must be poured into the ear, and left there till the next day, when syringing may be used.

Do not get into habit of putting cotton in ear—accumulations may eventually plug it.

REMOVING INSECTS FROM EAR

A teaspoon of warm olive oil, or camphorated oil poured into the ear and held there for a few minutes will destroy the bug and will easily pour out of the ear with the bug. If the insect remains in the ear, fill the ear with warm water, it will float out the oil and insect.

The instant an insect gets inside the ear, turn it to the sun. If this happens at night put patient in dark room and shine light in ear canal. Insects are generally attracted to light. A ripe apple or peach applied to the ear also attracts some type insects.

DEAFNESS CAUSED BY WAX ACCUMULATION

Take clean, fine black wool, dip it in civet, and put it into the ear; as it dries, which in a day or 2 it will, dip it again; and keep it moistened in the ear for 3 weeks or a month.
The American Family Receipt Book, 1854

Take an equal quantity of good Hungary water and oil of bitter almonds, beat them together, and drop 3 drops in the ears, going to bed; stop them with black wool, and repeat this 9 nights at least.

Place a small piece of cotton, upon which a little oil of almonds has been dropped, into the ear, and let it remain there for a day or two. Then syringe the ear with a little warm milk and water, or a solution of mild soap or with a solution of common salt and water in the proportion of 2 drachms of salt to ½ an ounce of water. The solution of salt is the best solvent of accumulated wax in the ear.
Practical Housekeeping, 1887

Sassafras oil 15 drops, glycerine 1½ drachms, olive oil ½ ounce may be dropped into the ear once or twice a day, a few drops at a time.

Melt the fat of a hedgehog and pour a drop into the ear at night. This relieves the eardrum and dissolves the hard wax which is the frequent cause of deafness. A good substitute for the hedgehog fat is the fat of the goose. Melt a little of this and drop a little of it, warm, in the ear when in bed, and sleep lying on the opposite ear. Next night do the other ear.

Obtain pickerel oil, and apply 4 drops morning and evening to the ear. Great care should be taken to obtain oil that is perfectly pure.

A drop of skunk oil in the ears is wonderful! I've used it for years.

L. E. O., 1963

Drop into the ear eel's oil, 2 or 3 drops, then stop the ear with fine wool, and repeat the dose until it cures.

Put the leaves of houseleek in a vial, place this inside of a loaf of bread-dough, and bake it along with the bread. It forms a soft, oil substance, which may be dropped into the ear every night, 1 or 2 drops at a time. It causes an indescribable, stimulating sensation.

J. King, 1864

Bruise, in a marble mortar, the flowers, leaves, and stalks, of fresh foxglove; and, mixing the juice with double the quantity of brandy, keep it for use. The herb flowers in June, and the juice will thus keep good till the return of that season. The method of using it is, to drop every night, in the ear, a single drop; then, moistening a bit of lint with a little of the juice, put that also into the ear, and take it out next morning, till the cure be completed.

Take the juice of sow-thistle, and heat it with a little oil of bitter almond, in the shell of a pomegranate, and drop some of it into the ears. It is a good remedy for deafness, singings, and other diseases of the head and ears.

P. F. Bowker, 1836

DEFICIENCY OF WAX

Deafness is sometimes the consequences of a morbidly dry state of the inner passages of the ear. In such cases, introduce a bit of cotton wool dipped in an equal mixture of oil of turpentine and oil of almonds, or in the liniment of carbonate of ammonia.

When the ear is very dry, and there is a deficiency of moisture the following may be used: glycerine 1 drachm, oil of turpentine ½ drachm, linseed oil ½ ounce.

RUNNING EARS

The ears may be syringed out with warm soap suds, after which an infusion of golden seal should be injected. A decoction of equal parts of golden seal and wild indigo root may be used in some cases.

ECZEMA

Wash the parts thoroughly with pure castile soap, and dry carefully; then apply borax and vaseline. To cure this disease radically a powerful blood purifier is needed.

Apply 2 ounces glycerine with a teaspoon of boracic acid dissolved in it. A sure cure and there is no danger of using too much.

Use freely a wash made with water and a little dissolved alum.

Add flour of sulfur to lard and use paste as salve.

Bathe parts with strong vinegar. [The strength of vinegar may be increased by boiling it.]

Rub parts with lemon.

Make poultice of fresh potato with a small quantity of camphor and apply.

Take beef bones, burn them in a fire till they become white, pound them fine, sift them, mix the powder with molasses; take it 3 times a day, before eating. Continue this for several days, take a cabbage stump, scrape out the inside, put it into cream and simmer it well. Anoint the part affected, this has been known to perform great and wonderful cures.

P. F. Bowker, 1836

First apply a poultice of wheat bread and milk, for 48 hours; then take 2 handfuls of strawberry leaves, celandine, and wood betony herb, of each ½ pint; hog's lard 2 pounds; and pine tar ½ pint; simmer the whole together 1 hour, and apply to the part affected. Such things as would cleanse the blood might also with propriety be given.

L. Sperry, 1843

Procure some strawberry leaves and lay the outside, or woolly side of the leaf on the parts affected. They must be laid very thick, and be changed occasionally. They will draw out the inflammation, and cure the disease.

*The Modern Home Cook Book
and Family Physician,* about 1880

Rub the hands with pure juice of poke berries and in a week they will be like a baby's for softness—the only sure remedy for the disease. Others relieve for a time, but this positively cures. It cools and soothes inflamed tissues.

Take berries of poke, and make an ointment by simmering them in fresh butter or lard. With this anoint the part affected frequently, which will seldom fail of curing.

Wash parts frequently with a strong decoction made of prince's pine herb.

Take 2 tablespoons hog lard, 1 large handful of cheese plant herb, and a small handful of cheese plant roots. Fry in lard till the lard looks green, then strain and stir until thick. You can add a teaspoon borax.

Apply oil of cade or juniper.

The juice of fresh watercress is said to have cured stubborn cases of eczema.

Boil the fresh corms of Indian turnip in hog's lard to make a strong ointment.

To 1 quart pure cider vinegar add 1 ounce of bloodroot. Shake well and let it stand a few hours. Bathe the parts affected 2 or 3 times a day until cured.

Steep an ounce each of bloodroot and yellow dock root in a pint of alcohol and ½ pint of vinegar. Apply to affected parts.

Take 2 teaspoons yellow dock root, 6 teaspoons poke root and 1 teaspoon hog lard. Mix in 1 pint of water boiled down to ½ pint. Apply.

INTERNAL AND EXTERNAL TREATMENTS

Take swamp sassafras bark [*Magnolia virginiana*], boil it in water very strong, take some of the water and wash the part affected; to the remainder of the water add hog's lard, and simmer it over a moderate fire till the water is gone. Anoint the part affected, after washing; (continue 4 days) never fails of a cure. A sirup for the above recipe. Take tag alder bark [*Alnus serrulata*], dwarf elder root [*Sambucus ebulus*], black cherry bark [*Prunus serotina*], buck-thorn bark [*Rhamnus cathartica*], equal quantities, boiled strong and sweetened with loaf sugar. Take a tablespoon 3 times a day. Take of sulphur 2 parts, cream of tartar 1 part, mix in molasses, take a teaspoon 3 mornings running, then miss 3, continue until taken 9 mornings, then miss 9, and go over the process again. For a wash, Epsom salts dissolved in soft water, wash the parts affected, with a linen cloth, 2 or 3 times a day. For a salve take cow-slips [*Primula veris*], 1 pailful; boil in fresh soft water until tender, skim out the herb and add to the liquor 1 teacup full of fresh lard, simmer to an oil; after washing with the salts, anoint the parts affected, and wear linen next the skin.

Dr. L. Sperry, 1843

Drink freely of a decoction made with root of burdock.

Drink 2 or 3 times a day an infusion made with equal parts sassafras, sarsaparilla, root of Rocky Mountain grape and wintergreen leaves.

Drink tea made of equal parts of yellow dock root, burdock root, poke root and sarsaparilla. Use one of the following as a lotion: tincture of bloodroot; witch hazel extract; liquid marigold or glycerine and lime water.

Take wild cherry bark, tag alder bark and green of elder, boil and add saltpeter the size of a walnut to a quart. Take 1 teaspoon morning and evening. Also use a teaspoon of saltpeter in a pint of water, as a wash.

Make a strong tea of elm bark; drink the tea freely; wash the affected part in the same; or, take 1 ounce of blue flag root, steep it in ½ pint of gin; take teaspoon 3 times a day; and wash with the same; or take

1 ounce of oil of tar, 1 drachm of oil of checkerberry; mix. Take from 5 to 20 drops, morning and night, as the stomach will bear.

ERYSIPELAS or ST. ANTHONY'S FIRE

Wash parts with a solution of boric acid, ½ teaspoon, to 8 teaspoons tepid water.

Put a tablespoon of baking soda in 1 pint of water and bathe parts several times a day.

Take of fine spirits of turpentine and highly rectified spirits of wine, equal parts, mix these well together, and keep it tight from the air. Anoint the affected part often with the composition, after shaking the bottle. Be a little careful not to approach the eyes. It can be done with a feather to the best advantage. After it has pretty much healed, anoint with mutton marrow. This serves to soften, and helps allay the inflammation.

Take camphor gum and hog lard, melt together. Apply to the affected part and cover with soft cloth. Generally 1 application will cure.

Letter, 1931

Sprinkling the body with fine starch, or with wheat flour, will greatly assist to cool and allay the irritation. A teaspoon of sugar of lead put in 3½ pints of cold water, and used as a remedy by washing the body, is also a valuable application.

Apply glycerine 2 or 3 times a day.

Keep parts well bathed with witch hazel extract.

Apply sour milk, buttermilk or whey to affected parts.

Make egg wine, rich and good for drinking; drink a part of it and wash the part affected with the other.

Dissolve 5 ounces of salt in 1 pint of good brandy, and take 2 tablespoons, 3 times a day.

Boil white navy beans until soft and apply them as poultice. Renew frequently.

Cut fine 2 onions and cook till tender in 1 pint of water. Thicken with wheat bran and add bicarbonate of soda the size of a bean. Change poultices as often as necessary, until inflammation is reduced.

Bloodroot is a specific for erysipelas.

Dr. Randale, 1852

The juice of fresh poke berries cures.

One pint of sweet milk and a handful of poke roots steeped and used as a local application is a sure cure.

Make an infusion of figwort herb. Drink it as a beverage and make a poultice of the herb to be applied to inflamed surfaces.

A strong decoction of sweet fern leaves applied externally, at the same time that it is taken freely internally, is considered by many to be peculiarly efficacious in curing many eruptions of the skin, particularly St. Anthony's fire, and poisoning from swamp sumac.

W. M. Hand, 1820

As a local application, slippery elm has been found efficacious. Make a mucilage of it, and apply it warm on cloths to the face.

One teacupful of the bark of the root of sumac [Rhus glabra], the same quantity of the twigs of sumac, pounded fine and 1 handful of double rose leaves [petals], 1 handful of green bark of elder [Sambucus canadensis], pounded fine, boiled for some time, in 2 quarts of water, strain and clear and boil it down to ½ pint; add 1 pound fresh butter, ½ ounce of Burgundy pitch, 1 ounce of Barbary tallow [wax of Myrica cerifera berries], and 4 ounces of white rosin, simmer it moderately on coals, stir it often till it is all melted down. Strain it again, and it is fit for use; equal to any salve ever made.

Dr. L. Sperry, 1843

Take equal quantities of wild lettuce [Lactuca canadensis], burdock root [Arctium lappa] and sweet elder bark [Sambucus canadensis] and boil them together. Let the patient drink freely of this liquor. Take likewise, ground hemlock [Taxus minor] and bittersweet [Solanum dulcamara], and boil them together strong, and bathe the whole body with this decoction.

J. Monroe, 1824

Stew cranberries until soft and apply as poultice. Whiskey added to poultice is more effective.

If the disease is located about the face and head, the parts affected should be steamed over a decoction of bitter herbs, as catnip, tansy, boneset, hops, etc., 2 or 3 times a day. In the mean time, apply over the affected parts a poultice of cranberries, made by boiling a pint or 2 of the berries, soft, allowing plenty of juice to remain; then take a teacupful, juice and berries, mash, and mix in a little powdered slippery elm, or a little wheat bran, spread thin on a cloth, and apply. Renew 2 or 3 times a day. If you should not be able to check the disease, and vesicles or blisters should form, and ulceration take place, you must poultice with slippery elm and hop yeast; and it would also be well to wash the ulcers with a decoction of the wild indigo leaves or root. The patient, during the whole treatment should drink freely of a tea made of burdock root, sassafras bark of root, and elder flowers.

EYES

INFLAMED, IRRITATED OR SORE

Let there be an occasional pressure of the finger on the ball of the eye, and let the pressure always be from the nose and toward temples. Wash eyes 3 times a day in cool water.

Borax, ½ drachm; camphor water, 3 ounces. This is unexcelled for the treatment of inflammation of the eyes. In using it lean back and drop 3 drops in the corner of each, and then open the eyes and let it work in. Use it as often as the eyes feel badly.

Thoroughly dissolve a heaped teaspoon of boracic acid in ½ pint of cold water. Then apply to the eyes with the fingers, never using a sponge or cloth. Let this solution dry on the eyelids. Use it before going to bed, and in the morning again.

When eyes become inflamed from any cause, do not rub them at all—such irritation is dangerous—but bathe them in tepid milk and water, keep the bowels open by some gentle medicine and eat little meat. The eyes are very sensitive to the state of the stomach. Avoid the glare of strong light.

Pare and quarter a potato, wash, dry and grate as fine as possible. Place between pieces of cambric [fine white linen] and put the poultice over the inflamed eye, keeping it there about 15 minutes.

Continue the operation 3 successive nights. Poultices made from mashed cooked beets or flaxseed meal are also good.

Take 3 eggs, and break them into 1 quart cold rainwater; stir until thoroughly mixed; bring to a boil on a slow fire, stirring often; add ½ ounce sulphate of zinc; continue the boiling for 2 minutes, then set it off; take the curd that settles at the bottom of this and apply to the eye at night with a bandage; strain the liquid through a cloth, and use for bathing the eyes occasionally. This is the best eyewater ever made for man or beast.

A poultice made with slippery elm powder applied to the eyes, in an inflammation is good, as there is no danger of injuring them by it.

Get the roots of linwood (some call it basswood), wash and scrape the outer bark clean, then scrape the inner bark very fine, filling a tumbler about ⅓ full. Then fill the tumbler nearly full of rainwater. It will, in a little while, thicken like jelly. Now take a thin, soft cloth, the thinner the better, put some of the mucilage between 2 pieces and place it upon the eyes. It is very soothing.

Get some cheese plant leaves and roots, boil them till soft, then use the infusion to bathe the eyes. Bind the boiled leaves and roots on the eyes. In a few hours the redness is gone.

Old letter

The seeds of quince soaked in warm water afford a soothing lotion for inflamed eyes.

Take of the limbs and twigs of sassafras, and steep a strong decoction, which must be strained and a portion of mare's milk added to it. Use as a wash.

Fresh elder leaves laid over the eyes and held in place with bandage clears the eyes and brow.

B. F. S., M.D., 1912

Take of green ozier, the bark scraped fine, 1 ounce; add 3 gills of soft water; infuse or steep them a few minutes, and wet the eyes affected, with this infusion, several times a day, applied either warm or cold.

Take blue violets which are growing wild in most places, dig them up, top and root, wash clean, dry them and make a tea; drink several times a day, wetting the eyes each time, and it will soon cure.

A few drops of cajuput oil poured on a bit of soft linen cloth, and suffered to evaporate while held close to the afflicted organs of sight, over which the cloth is afterward to remain tied all night, has proved highly serviceable.

There is nothing better than a poultice of cold tea grounds. Renew it when it gets warm or dry.

Moisten pads of cloth with witch hazel and apply to the closed eyes.

A very good eye-water may be made by steeping the leaves which remain on the beech tree during the winter, and applying it cold, by means of a rag, to the eye.

A squaw's cure. Take rattlesnake plantain, 1 handful, the same quantity of lobelia, steep it in 1 quart of water 24 hours, then strain and bottle it, and it is fit for use, wash 3 times a day; it will cure.

Take ½ pound of camomile, and 1 quart of new milk; boil it down to a pint; add ½ pint West India rum, put in 4 ounces of loaf sugar, and it is fit for use. Bathe the parts affected 3 or 4 times a day.

The Indians in the Midwest considered golden seal a specific for sore or inflamed eyes. A wash was made by boiling about a teaspoon of the dried root in about a cup of water for several minutes. Strain and use when cool.

C. S. Rafinesque, 1828

Take 1 teacupful of green elder and the bark of the roots of sumac, equal parts; 1 handful of double rose leaves [petals], and live-forever, equal parts; pound them fine, put them into 2 quarts of water, and boil for 20 minutes, strain off and boil down to ½ a pint; then add 1 pint of sweet cream, and 4 ounces of clear rosin, set it on the coals, and stir it until it melts down to an oil; strain it again, and it is fit for use.

EYEWASHES

Bathe in hot water, never using cold; and neither children or adults should use water below 50° temperature in washing, as cold water is very injurious to the eyes.

Bathe eyes with soft water, or slightly diluted witch hazel.

Take equal parts of rosewater and witch hazel. Apply to the eyes as often as necessary.

Spirits of camphor reduced a little with water, soak a rag with it and hold it on the outside of the lids. Be careful not to get it in the eyes.

A weak solution of ordinary tea may be used as an eyewash.

Witch hazel leaves, golden seal root, equal parts, steeped in water, and a little alum added.

Make a wash with equal parts of golden seal root and alum root.

Make a strong tea of equal parts of hyssop leaves and St. John's wort leaves and flowers. Apply this to the eyes on cloths, or by letting a few drops fall in the eyes, 2 or 3 times a day.

BLACK OR BRUISED EYE

Immediately apply a cloth wet with water, just as hot as can be borne. Keep this up 20 minutes, and the treatment will prevent discoloration.

Apply raw beef steak to bruised eye.

Boil a handful of hyssop leaves in a little water, till they are quite tender; then put them up in linen, apply it hot to the eye, tie it on tightly at bedtime, and the eye will next day be quite well.

Use a decoction of the roots of soapwort as poultice to remove discoloration.

Apply mashed fresh roots of Solomon's seal or a poultice of slippery elm.

FOREIGN MATTER IN THE EYE

Take a single [whole] flaxseed or seed of cleareye, moisten it on the tongue and put it under the lid; close the eye for a moment and the substance will adhere to the seed and come out with it.

Immerse the eye in cool [not cold] water, then wink and roll the eyeball until specks of dirt are removed.

STIES

Put a teaspoonful of black tea in a small bag, pour on it enough boiling water to moisten it; then put it on the eye pretty warm. Keep it on all night, and in the morning the sty will most likely be gone; if not, a second application is certain to remove it.

Put 1 teaspoon saleratus on a 3 inch square piece of muslin, fold so that the soda cannot fall out, and before going to sleep dip this muslin in water, lay it on the eye and fasten in place by means of a thin cheese cloth bandage. This will drive away unripe sties before morning. If the sty has come to a head, break open with a needle sterilized in a flame, and bathe the eye in warm bicarbonate of soda water, which may be followed by the application of a little vaseline.

Bathe eyes in warm boracic water, and then, splash with cold until they sting.

WEAK EYES

Bathe eyes night and morning in a tolerable strong solution of salt and water. Remarkable cures have been effected by this simple remedy. After bathing the eyes daily for about a week, intermit a day or 2, and then resume the daily bathing, and so on till your eyes get strong again.

Take rose petals, the more the better, and put them into a little water; then boil; after this strain it into a bottle and cork it tight. You will find this liquid very beneficial in removing redness and weakness from the eyes.

Cut a slice of stale bread as thin as possible; toast both sides well but don't burn; when cold, lay in cold spring or ice water; put between a piece of old linen and apply, changing when it gets warm.

Take ½ ounce of golden seal, pour ½ pint boiling water upon it and let cool. Bathe the eyes with a linen rag dipped in this, each night on going to bed, and you will soon effect a cure.

Three or 5 grains of alum dissolved in ½ pint of water, and applied to the eyes whenever they are weak or inflamed.

The eyes well washed with an infusion made with eyebright herb 2 or 3 times daily, or little pieces of linen dipped into it, and fastened over the eyes by means of a bandage during the night, will cleanse the eyes, make them clear, and strengthen the sight.

The juice or distilled water of eyebright herb taken inwardly, in white wine, or put into the eyes, is good for all things that cause dimness of sight; or it may be taken in a powder of the dried herb, mixed with a little sugar, mace and fennel seed; has a powerful effect to help and restore sight, decayed through age, and has been known to restore sight to those who have been nearly blind.

Purple loosestrife infusion of the herb used as a wash is one of the best remedies for preserving the sight, and for the cure of sore eyes. It is fully as valuable as eyebright. It will cure blindness, provided the crystalline humor be not injured or destroyed.

Mrs. A. Matteson, 1894

Take the pith from the stalk of a sassafras bush, mix it with a little water, about blood warm. Wash the eyes 3 or 4 times a day. This is far superior to the celebrated eye water. Keep clear of greasy victuals.

When the sight is weak, but with no special disease present, it may be very much improved by one of the following methods: Take a handful of fresh red peppers, or ginger root, and pour over them a ½ pint of pure alcohol. Wipe twice daily the brow above the eye and the temple with a little of this on a soft sponge, and let it dry. Or take a heaping tablespoonful of clean rock salt, and let it dissolve in a quart of rain water. Immerse the face in this every morning, and open the eyes while under the water so the salt can act directly on the organ. This latter is most excellent also in cases of redness of the eyes.

Personal Beauty, by D. Brinton,
M.D., and G. Naphey, M.D., 1870

WEEPING EYES

Use a wash at night and morning of common table salt, and water.

Apply a poultice made of elder flowers.

Apply a poultice made of slippery elm bark.

Wash eyes morning and night with decoction made of chamomile flowers.

Make a strong decoction of chamomile, boiled in sweet milk. Bathe the eyes with this several times a day, as warm as can be suffered. If this remedy is persevered in for a length of time, it is most certain to effect a cure. It may be necessary to follow this treatment for 6 or 8 weeks; but this would be nothing if you only come off conqueror at last.

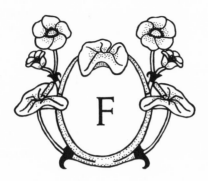

FAINT

Effusion of cold water on the face, stimulants to the nostrils, pure air, and recumbent position.

Rub the soles of one that has fainted or is unconscious—this will bring him to at once.

A hearty sneeze is said to have the effect of warding off a threatening fainting spell. A grain or 2 of pepper, snuff or tobacco introduced into the nose, or tickling the interior of the nose a little with a feather, will usually insure a sneeze. The sneezing stimulates the blood vessels of the brain. It is handy to know this, when smelling salts and other means are absent.

Apply fresh pennyroyal herb to the nostrils with vinegar.
                                        Elias Smith, Physician, 1826

Oil of pennyroyal with vinegar.

Take of oil of lavender, 6 ounces; oil of rosemary, 2 ounces; cinnamon, 1 ounce; cloves, 2 drachms; nutmeg, ½ ounce; red sanders in shavings, 3 drachms; alcohol, 4 pounds. Dissolve 10 days and filter. This is a grateful cordial for relieving languor and faintness. From 10 to a 100 drops may be conveniently taken dropped on sugar.

Chew sassafras bark of root when feeling faint.

FATIGUE

When very weary or weak from exhaustion, heat some milk to scalding point, then sip it as hot as possible. It refreshes almost instantly.

How often we hear women who do their own work say that by the time they have prepared a meal, and it is ready for the table they are too tired to eat. One way to mitigate this evil is to take, about ½ hour before dinner, a raw egg, beat it until light, put in a little sugar, flavor it and drink it down. It will remove the faint, tired out feeling, and will not spoil your appetite for dinner.

Mrs. M. W. Ellsworth, 1897

FEET

ATHLETE'S FOOT

Apply jell of Aloe vera.

Apply whale oil. Mask odor of this oil with a little oil of cloves.

BUNIONS

Put a little pulverized saltpeter in olive oil; shake well, and rub on inflamed joints night and morning, and more frequently, if painful.

COLD FEET

Every night on going to bed, dip the feet in shallow, cold water, 2 or 3 times, then rub briskly with a coarse towel till dry; then take hold of each end of the towel and draw it back and forth through the hollow of the foot until a glow is excited.

Raise the body on the toes for a minute or 2, then drop quickly to the heels, then stand again on the toes and continue changing until the blood goes tingling through the feet and warms them up.

CORNS

Take 1 teaspoon pine tar, 1 teaspoon coarse brown sugar, and 1 teaspoon saltpeter; the whole to be warmed together. Spread it on kip leather the size of the corns, and in 2 days they will be drawn out.

Wash and dry the foot thoroughly, put on a sprinkling of dry sulphur night and morning for several weeks, and a cure is assured.

Equal parts of muriatic acid and nitric acid. Take a sharp pointed stick and dip in the acid and touch up the corns and they will turn yellow and rot out.

Soft corns may be relieved by dissolving a piece of ammonia, the size of a large bean, in 1 ounce of water, and applying the solution as hot as can be borne.

Applying strong acetic acid night and morning will usually effect a cure.

Bathe foot or feet well in warm water, about ½ hour before going to bed. When the corns have become soft from bathing, shave down the horny parts smooth, but not so close as to produce blood. Then moisten the tops of them with spittle, and rub over them a little lunar caustic. This must be gently rubbed on, until a sufficiency of it sticks on the corns, to change them to a dark gray color, and next to a deep black. Put a little cotton over them, to prevent the stocking from rubbing them, and in a few days they will come out by the roots.

Boil tobacco down to an extract, then mix with it a quantity of white pine pitch; apply it to the corn, renewing it once a week until corn disappears.

Soak foot in hot mustard and water, rubbing the corn all the time. In most cases it can be picked out from the heart. An application of strong vinegar will help the operation, while, if obstinate, touch with iodine every other day, never neglecting the nightly bath.

Take bark of the common willow, burn to ashes, mix them with strong vinegar and apply to the parts. This is a very effectual remedy for corns or warts.

Dr. R. L. Louis, 1877

Make a paste of hickory ashes and strong vinegar. Apply to the corns.

A small application of beef tallow on the hard substance around corns will in due time make them soft again.

Take ¼ cup of strong vinegar, crumb into it some bread. Let stand ½ hour, or until it softens into a good poultice. Then apply, on retiring at night. In the morning the soreness will be gone, and the corn can be picked out. If the corn is a very obstinate one, it may require 2 or more applications to effect a cure.

Soak an onion in vinegar several hours, then cut in two and bind 1 section on the corn at night. The core can generally be picked out in the morning. Repeat if necessary.

Use a salve made of equal parts of roasted onions and soft soap; apply it hot. Or apply a sponge wet with a solution of pearlash.

Take a small piece of flannel which has not been washed, wrap or sew it round the corn and toe. One thickness will be sufficient. Wet the flannel where the corn is, night and morning, with fine sweet oil. Renew the flannel weekly, and at the same time pare the corn, which will very soon disappear.

Apply a little cotton wool soaked in castor oil. Bind it upon the corn with a strip of soft, old linen.

Apply oil of sassafras to corns.

Apply oil of wintergreen for soft corns.

Spread a plaster of white pine turpentine, put it on the corn, let it stay till it comes off of its own accord. Repeat this 3 times, and it will effect a cure.

Thrusting the toe into a lemon, to be kept on overnight, will make the removal of a corn easy; 2 or 3 applications will suffice for the worst cases.

The juice squeezed out of the fresh plant of celandine herb will cure if applied.

Take nightshade berries; boil them in hog's lard and anoint the corn with the salve. It will not fail to cure.

A root [corm] of wild Indian turnip, scraped and bound upon the corn, after the corn has been cut and made tender, will cure it in a short time.

INGROWN TOENAILS

Soak the foot in warm water and soap for ¼ hour, until the nail becomes soft and pliable, then, with a sharp knife, scrape the nail quite thin on its upper surface. This will cause it to flatten out in growing and to assume its proper shape.

Dip a rag in a strong solution of tannic acid and water, and place between the nail and inflamed parts of the toe. This treatment persevered in, should bring relief.

Make a salve of common laundry soap, a little cream and pulverized sugar. Apply morning and night until relieved.

ITCHING FEET

Take any kind of tallow, tallow the part affected, and rub it in by a hot fire, on going to bed. Repeat it 3 or 4 times.

PERSPIRING FEET

To prevent the unpleasantness, place oatmeal or bran in the socks, or sprinkle socks with a powder made of equal parts of fuller's earth, powdered starch and powdered zinc.

SWOLLEN FEET

Take wheat bran, mix in some soda, put it in a bucket and bathe and soak your feet. Repeat for a week.

Soak the feet in vinegar each night until relieved. This will cure swelling or an extremely tired feeling in the feet, or perspiration. The vinegar may be diluted if very strong.

Take plantain leaves (which can be found in almost any grass plot, and in public parks); wilt them by putting separately between the hands; cover the swollen parts with them, and keep in place by wrapping the limb with rags or a towel on going to bed at night, or keep them on during the day if not obliged to be upon the feet. A cure will be speedily effected.

TENDER AND ACHING FEET

Use water as hot as can be borne. Baths of sand, warm and moist, are also good. Bury the feet in this up to the ankles, and let remain from 20 to 30 minutes, keeping the sand warm by adding hot water occasionally.

Make a strong decoction of white oak bark or red oak bark, and soak feet night and morning.

Take a large leaf of horseradish, burdock, cabbage, or mullein; cut out the hard fibers that run through the leaf; place it on a hot shovel for a moment to soften it, fold it, and fasten it closely in the hollow of the foot by cloth bandage.

Roast onions until quite soft; peel off the outside, mash them, and apply on a cloth bandage.

FELON or WHITLOW

Dip the finger quickly into boiling water several times in succession. This may be done without risk of scalding. Repeat every hour for several hours, and the cure is generally complete.

When you fear a felon is coming, put 1 pint boiling water on the back of the stove, add 1 teaspoon saleratus and 1 wineglass vinegar. Hold your finger in this as hot as can be borne. Reheat and repeat about every ½ hour, till all the matter has been drawn to 1 place, then open the felon with a sterilized, sharp knife, remove the foreign matter and clean and bandage.

Immerse the part in tepid water of agreeable temperature, as frequently and as long as possible; dress with a poultice of soft boiled carrots. Touch occasionally with a stimulating oil.

Apply a poultice of raw onions, and change every 6 hours.

Procure several lemons. Cut a small opening in the end of 1 and push the finger in. Keep it there until the lemon ceases to draw, then apply another, and keep on until the pain is relieved.

Take common rock salt, as used for salting down pork or beef, dry in an oven, then pound it fine and mix with spirits of turpentine in equal parts; put it in a rag and wrap it around the parts affected; as it gets dry put on more, and in 24 hours you are cured.

Take a teaspoon of fine salt, a tablespoon of black pepper, a tablespoon of vinegar and the yolk of an egg, simmer together and bind on. Renew twice a day. A never failing remedy.

Take 1 pound of mutton tallow, 1 tablespoon black pepper, 1 tablespoon of saltpeter, ½ a spoonful Scotch snuff, 1 spoonful of spirits of turpentine, a piece of verdigris, as large as a walnut; simmer it together until it is well mixed. Strain it through flannel, and it is fit for use. Apply it to part affected and wind on flannel. It is a great salve and will cure the pain of a felon, in 2 hours after it is applied.

Put wood ashes, covered with warm water in a dish on the stove, hold the affected part in this, allowing it to get as hot as can be borne.

Get a pitch-pine knot from an old log, the side next to, or in the ground, split the knot fine, boil out ½ pound of pitch; take 4 ounces of strong tobacco, boil the liquor, simmer it over a moderate heat, stir it all the time till it forms a salve altogether. Lay the plaster on the wrist if the tumor is on the hand or fingers; if on the foot or toes, lay the plaster on ankle; or wherever it may be, lay it above the next joint. This will take out all the pain in a short time. Dress the sore with any other proper salve. This cure is infallible.

Dr. L. Sperry, 1843

Carry the hand in a sling, and apply a leech.

C. Kinsley, 1876

Wet powdered sassafras bark of root in cold water for a poultice. Keep it wet with cold water.

Bind up the finger in cloth and keep it wet with oil of spike, until all soreness is gone.

Apply the bruised leaves of smartweed and bind on tight as can be borne.

Take 1 pound of yellow dock root, boil it in 2 quarts of water, down to 1 pint; then thicken it with Indian meal, and apply it to the part affected.

Take of blue flag root, and white hellebore equal parts, and boil them in milk and water; hold the finger in this as hot as can be borne about 15 minutes, then lay the hot roots on the felon about 1 hour, and it will soon disappear.

Take the outer bark of white birch, boil it in new milk, until the liquor is very strong, and apply it to the part affected.

Take wild red cherry bark, quite a quantity of it, and boil it down to a salve, and apply it to the parts affected, and it will in most cases cure.

Recipe from Seneca Indians

Take an earthen crock, put in a quantity of live coals, throw on a handful each of hops, rye flour, and brown sugar; then steam the affected part for about 15 minutes, repeating 2 or 3 times, by holding it over the vessel. The better way is to bore a hole through a board, thus having the affected part only coming in contact with the steam. This is guaranteed as a certain cure.

Take the root [corm] of Jack-in-the-pulpit, either green or dry; grate about ½ teaspoon into 4 tablespoons of sweet milk; simmer gently a few minutes, then thicken with bread crumbs, and apply hot as possible. This can be heated again 2 or 3 times, adding a little milk each time. If the felon is just starting, this will drive it back; if somewhat advanced, it will draw it out quickly and gently. It is well to put a little tallow on the poultice, especially after opening, to prevent sticking. This same poultice is good for a carbuncle or any other rising.

C. H. Fowler, W. H. DePuy, 1880

The juice of the leaves of true love, applied to felons, or those nails, or sores, gathered at the roots of them, will heal them in a short time.

Make a poultice of equal parts of powdered slippery elm bark, poke root, blue flag, and lobelia seeds, mix with hot lye, and change twice a day.

When the felon first appears, procure some poke root, and roast a piece sufficient to cover your finger. When it is roasted tender, cut it open and bind it on the felon as hot as can be borne; repeat this when the root becomes dry, until the pain subsides. If the felon is too far advanced to put back, this same remedy will hasten it on and cure it in a few days, as it softens the skin.

As soon as the parts begin to swell, wrap the part affected in a cloth thoroughly saturated with tincture of lobelia, and the felon is dead. It never fails if applied in season.

Whitlow grass is held to be exceedingly good for those imposthumes in the joints and under the nails, which are called whitlows, felons, andicons and nailwheels, by physicians.

FEMALE WEAKNESS

Heart's ease herb, spikenard root, a small part of bloodroot, turkey root, wild licorice, a few roots of white pond lilies, a good parcel of female flowers. It often grows by the side of ponds, and has a leaf and blossoms some like cowslips; but it grows single, 1 root or stalk by itself, and some smaller than the cowslip; the leaves are green and the blossom is yellow. This is one of the finest roots for the use of females in the world. Use double the quantity of this and equal parts of the others, make a sirup of them, boil them in fair water until the substance is out; strain it off, sweeten it with honey, add as much rum to it as will keep it from souring. Drink ½ gill on going to bed every night. This will strengthen the system, and throw off all obstructions. It is best for persons so complaining, to wear a thick piece of flannel on the small of the back.

Dr. L. Sperry, 1843

Take 3 quarts of strong vinegar, 2 ounces anvil scales, pound fine and the dust blown out, 1 pugil of Virginia or Seneca snakeroot, 1 pugil of mountain dittany, or garden ground ivy, simmer them together in an iron pot to a pint; put into it 10 grains of myrrh and 10 grains of aloes, a pound of sugar and a gill of spirits; cover it close, and simmer it down on coals to thick molasses, and put it by for use. A teaspoon is a dose, night, morning and night; then miss the like times, and take it again; and so continue the course till nature is braced and strengthened. This is a cure for obstructed menses, or wasting fluor. With this medicine many have been relieved: the barren have become fruitful; and those despairing of life, have been restored to health.

P. Smith, 1812

Take the following in powder form; 1 ounce cranesbill root, 2 ounces white poplar bark, 1 ounce bistort root, 1 ounce golden seal root, ½ ounce cinnamon, ½ ounce cloves, ¼ ounce ginger, ½ pound sugar. Mix. Dose of the powder, is a teaspoon in ½ cup of boiling water, 3 times a day; drink the clear only.

Take of cranesbill root 4 ounces, comfrey root 4 ounces, beth-root, orange peel 1 ounce, cinnamon ½ ounce, well pounded and infused in 3 quarts of good wine, and sweetened with honey. This is very useful in cases of debility, fluor-albus, and immoderate flow of the menses. For a dose, ½ wineglass 3 times a day.

Take ¼ pound of comfrey root, dried, 2 ounces of elecampane root and 1 ounce of hoarhound; boil from 3 quarts to 3 pints of soft water, strain and add while warm, ½ ounce of beth-root, pulverized; also, a pint of brandy and a pound of loaf sugar. Dose, from ½ to ⅔ wineglassful 3 or 4 times a day.

Another good medicine is Solomon's seal and life-of-man root, made in a sirup and sweetened with honey.

One ounce black cherry bark, 1 ounce of butternut bark, and 4 ounces of the bark of rose willow bark, boil in 4 quarts of soft water, add 1 quart Madeira wine, and 6 ounces loaf sugar, strain, and it is fit for use; take 1 wineglass 3 times a day before eating. Omit at particular circumstances [during menstrual period]. Or boil 1 pound rose willow bark, in 6 quarts of water to 3, add 3 pints of port wine, and 4 ounces of loaf sugar. Dose 1 wineglassful 3 times a day.

To 1 quart of good whiskey add the following: pleurisy root, blue cohosh root, black cohosh, each, in coarse powder, 1 tablespoon; balm of gilead buds, tamarac, angelica root, each in coarse powder, 2 teaspoons; bloodroot in coarse powder, 1 teaspoon; mix; let it stand 10 or 12 days, shaking frequently. The dose is a teaspoon 3 times a day, gradually increased, as the stomach can bear it, to 1 or 2 tablespoons; it should be taken in sweetened water. This is a most excellent medicine.

J. King, M.D., 1855

I'll guarantee any woman good health and no miscarriages if she will try this. Take 3 teaspoons crow corn root and steep it in 1 pint of whiskey ½ hour and take 1 teaspoon squaw root and steep in ½ cup of boiling water ½ hour. Then strain both and put into a 1 pint whiskey bottle and if it isn't quite full, fill to top with boiled water just so you have 1 pint when all is done. Take 1 teaspoon at a dose 2 or 3 times a day according to your weakness. I have no more awful cramps like I had when I used to flow.

Mrs. E. M. Cook, 1916

Excellent for the whites and a superior female tonic. Take star root, gentian root, black-root, each 1 ounce finely powdered. Steep for 30 or 40 minutes in 1 pint of boiling water. When cold strain and put in a bottle adding 1 pint of port wine or gin. Dose, wineglassful 3 times a day.

J. H. McGirt, 1916

A very excellent tonic preparation for females to take, who are laboring under the whites, is the following: Take of golden seal, black cohush, colombo, ginseng, each, in coarse powder 1 ounce; boiling water 2 pints; mix, and then let them stand in a covered vessel till cold. Add 2 pints of whisky, and let it stand 5 or 6 days, frequently shaking. Then sweeten with white sugar to suit the taste. Dose, 2 tablespoons 3 or 4 times a day.

J. King, M.D., 1864

Take of comfrey root, Solomon's seal root, helonias each, bruised 1 ounce; chamomile flowers, colombo, gentian, cardamon, sassafras, each bruised ½ ounce. Let these articles macerate for 24 hours in sufficient boiling water to cover them, keeping them closely covered; then add sherry wine, 4 pints. Macerate for 14 days, express and strain. Dose, is from ½ to 2 fluid ounces, 3 or 4 times a day.

FEVERS

AGUE, MALARIAL, INTERMITTENT FEVER

Several remedies are employed against fever: the Jesuit's bark was formerly a certain one, but at present it has not always this effect, though they sell it genuine, and for the very best. Many people accuse it of leaving something noxious in the body. Yet it was commonly observed that when the bark was good, and it was taken as soon as the fever made its appearance, and before the body was weakened, it was almost sure to conquer the fever, so that the cold fits never returned, and no pain or stiffness remained in the limbs; but when the disease is rooted in, and has considerably weakened the patients, or they are naturally very weak, the fever leaves them after using the Jesuit's bark, but returns again in a fortnight's time, and obliges them to take the bark again; but the consequence is a pain and a stiffness in their limbs, and sometimes in their bowels, which almost hinders them from walking: this pain continues for several years together, and even accompanies some to the grave.

This bad effect is partly attributed to the bark, which can seldom be got genuine here, and partly to the little care which the patients take in using the bark. A man of my acquaintance was particularly dexterous in expelling the ague by the use of the Jesuit's bark. His manner of proceeding was as follows: when it was possible, the patient must use the remedy as soon as the fever has begun, and before it has settled in his body: but before he took the medicine, he was to take a diaphoretic remedy, as that had been found very salutary; and as the fever is frequently of such a nature here, as not to make the patient sweat, even when the hot fit is upon him, a perspiration was to be brought about by some other means. To that purpose the patient took his dose on the day he had his cold fit, and was not allowed to eat anything at night. The next morning he continued in a warm bed, drank a quantity of tea, and was well covered, that he might perspire plentifully. He continued so till the perspiration ceased, and then left the bed in a hot room, and washed his body with milk-warm water, in order to cleanse it from the impurities that settled upon it from the perspiration, and to prevent their stopping up the pores. The patient was then dried again, and at last he took the bark several times in one day. This was repeated twice or thrice on the days after he had the ague, and it commonly left him without returning, and most people recover so well, that they do not look pale after their sickness.

The bark of the root of the tulip tree, or *Liriodendron tulipifera,* taken in the same manner as the Jesuit's bark, sometimes had a similar effect.

Several people peeled the roots of the *Cornus florida,* or dogwood, and gave this peel to patients; and even some people, who could not be cured by the Jesuit's bark, have recovered by the help of this. I have likewise seen people cured of the fever, by taking brimstone reduced to powder, and mixed with sugar, every night before they went to bed, and every morning before they got up: they took it 3 or 4 times in the intervals, and at each time drank some warm liquor, to wash the powder down. However, others that tried the same remedy did not find much relief from it.

Some people collected the yellow bark of the peach tree, especially that which is on the root, and boiled it in water, till ½ of it was evaporated by boiling. Of this decoction the patient took every morning about a wineglassful, before he had eaten anything. This liquor has a disagreeable taste, and contracts the mouth and tongue like alum; yet several persons at Raccoon who had tried many remedies in vain, were cured by this.

Others boiled the leaves of the *Potentilla reptans,* or of the *Potentilla canadensis,* in water, and made the patients drink it before the ague fits came on, and it is well known that several persons have recovered by this means.

The people who are settled upon the river Mohawk in New York, both Indians and Europeans, collect the root of the *Geum rivale,* and pound it. This powder some of them boil in water till it is a pretty strong decoction: others only infuse cold water on it and leave it so for a day; others mix it with brandy. Of this medicine the patient is to take a wineglassful on the morning of the day when the fever does not come, before he has eaten anything. I was assured that this was one of the surest remedies, and more certain than the Jesuit's bark.

P. Kalm, 1772

Boneset or ague weed is a valuable remedy in all intermittent and remittent fevers—always acting as powerfully and beneficially as Peruvian bark. In fact, I think, in many cases, preferable to the bark, because it can be given when there is considerable fever: in which condition of a patient, the bark cannot be administered without great danger. For this reason also—I mean because it never increases fully, [it is used] not only in remitting bilious fever, but in typhus and yellow fevers. Dr. S. H. Hopkins of New Jersey, a physician of much celebrity, in an extensive practice of several years during which intermittent and typhus fevers were very prevalent, gave the boneset freely in warm decoction, with great success. By giving the boneset very copiously, he always produced sweating to allay the fever; and in dangerous cases, pushed the remedy so far as to produce emesis or vomiting—and also purging. He related to several of his friends that, many of the farmers in his vicinity, without calling in a physician, had, by the liberal use of a strong preparation of the boneset tea, given warm, entirely succeeded in curing themselves and their families, of both intermittent and typhus fevers. The truth is, that in low typhus, which is very dangerous, and always attended with an unusually dry and hot skin, the boneset is an inestimable remedy.

It is always used with the best effect, in a warm decoction of the flowers and leaves, which ought to be dried in the shade, and kept for use: the warm decoction is generally preferable to the plant in substance; and from 1 to 2 tablespoons, given every ½ hour, will in most cases, produce sweating without causing so much nausea of the stomach as to induce vomiting. If the fever is broken, and you wish to give strength to your patient, give the boneset in the powdered leaves and flowers, from 20 grains to a drachm, from 3 to 6 times in the lapse of 24 hours.

Boneset or ague weed has been used in the hospitals of New York with great success, given either as a tea or in powder.

J. C. Gunn, M.D., 1830

Take a good handful of cockleburs, put in a quart of water and simmer down to a pint. Take a small whisky glassful every 30 minutes until fever is broken. This has been tried in severe cases.

Mrs. A. M. M.

The leaves or flowers or both of a peach tree made into a strong tea, and a gill taken every hour until it acts well on the stomach, bowels and skin, will give great results in bilious fever. Take for several days until relief is obtained.

Mrs. E. E. J., 1916

Four ounces of galangal root in a quart of gin, steeped in a warm place; take often.

Miss E. N., 1890

An infusion of elder flowers is good for feverishness in children.

One ounce of Peruvian bark, 2 teaspoons of Virginia snakeroot, 2 teaspoons of cloves, 2 teaspoons sal soda, or salts of tartar all finely powdered, and mixed. Divide into 12 equal parts. Take 3 times (1 part each time) a day in water, or a glass of port wine.

Make a strong decoction of tansy herb and flowers steeped in white wine or whisky. Drink a teaspoon 3 times a day until cured.

EXTERNAL APPLICATIONS FOR CHILLS OF FEVER

Mix table salt up with dried hops and put into small bags. Heat bags and apply heated bags to the soles of feet and to wrists. Keep changing bags as they cool off until fever is broken.

Apply a poultice of fresh horseradish leaves to the soles of the feet. Pound the leaves to a pulp-like consistency. Place on gauze or linen, and apply to the soles of the feet; hold in place with bandage.

Mustard mixed with the white of an egg, and laid on the wrists, is beneficial in checking an ague fit. Put them on as soon as the first symptoms appear.

Take onions, slice them and apply to the soles of the feet. It will draw out high fever.

Potatoes, peeled and sliced, bound on the feet of children in high fever has reduced the fever at once.

DRINKS FOR FEVER

A decoction of the fruit of gooseberry bush is a very cooling and salutary drink in fevers.

Raspberries or strawberries quench thirst and abate heat, and strengthen the stomach.

The ripe berries of barberry contain a very acid red juice, which forms a pleasant and very useful drink in flux, and malignant fevers, for abating heat, quenching thirst, raising the strength, and preventing putrefaction.

Hulled barley grain makes a wholesome diet in fevers, and many other disorders; being more cooling and less cloying than any other grain.

There is no more refreshing drink than weak green tea, with lemon juice added instead of milk. It may be taken either cold or hot, but the latter is preferable.

Mix 1 part cider vinegar, 2 parts honey, 3 parts water.

The stomach will bear a great deal more of an infusion made of life-everlasting without inconvenience, than it will of water. Hence it is a useful drink in the early stages of fevers and colds.

A tea made of the twigs of fever-bush makes a pleasant and cooling drink.

The fresh dried herb of lemon balm made into a tea is good and very cooling.

The leaves of five-finger grass made into a tea is also very cooling.

The leaves and wood of sorrel tree are a fine astringent acid, refreshing, cooling, allaying thirst, and antifebrile. Clayton says that a decoction of the leaves mitigates the ardor of fevers, and helps their cure.

Put into a stone jug a little sage tea, 2 sprigs of fresh balm, and a small quantity of wood sorrel, having first washed and dried them. Peel thin a small lemon, and clear from the white; slice it and put in a bit of the peel. Then pour in 3 pints of boiling water, sweeten, and cover it close.

ALLEGED FEVER PREVENTIVES

The young shoots from poke plant taken in the spring when tender and cooked for greens once a year will keep the typhoid fever away. The greens must be parboiled or they will poison you.

Letter, 1931

A tea made of the roots of common elder is very good to prevent bilious fever.

Biting arsmart removes obstructions, helps the gravel; and in recent colds, is not exceeded by any other herb yet discovered. It is likewise a great preventive of fevers, if administered in season.

Cucumber tree [*Magnolia acuminata*] strengthens the stomach and nerves, warms and purifies the blood. The bark prepared in a tea or bitters, guards against the ague.

In early times—before physicians were so numerous—an infusion of the brittle spicy twigs of fever-bush or spice-bush was much used as a popular remedy, and even as a preventive of the fevers which attacked the first settlers.

W. Darlington, M.D., 1860

Those who are exposed by attending the sick, or where fevers or fluxes are suspected to be infectious, ought to take the butternut pills as a preventive. [Butternut pills were much used in folk medicine as a cathartic. See recipes under "Constipation."]

FEVER SORES

Take ½ pound of rosin, ½ pound beeswax, ½ pound lard, 2 ounces of oyster shells, burn them to lime, pulverize it fine, sift it through a fine cloth, put the whole into a kettle, simmer it over a moderate fire, then strain it, stir it until cold, then spread a plaster and apply it to the sore. Bathe and soak 3 times a day with buttermilk, to keep inflammation out. This is a certain cure, and is from the Seneca tribe of Indians.

Dr. L. Sperry, 1843

To stop a fever sore from coming to head, sweat it with flannel cloths dipped in hot brine. The cloths must be changed as often as they are cold, for 3 hours, then wash in brandy, and wrap in flannel, repeat it 3 or 4 times.

Take a quantity of the bark of sumach root and boil for 2 hours; strain and add fresh lard to the liquid. Then boil till the water is all out. Apply as a salve 3 times a day. Also good for minor cuts and bruises.

Kentucky recipe

Make a strong decoction of red clover flowers and apply to fever sores 3 or 4 times daily.

FLU, INFLUENZA, GRIPPE

Make a tea of red pepper or cayenne and take a tablespoon in a cup of hot water, drink slowly, before each meal and on retiring.

Take a bottle of alcohol and put in enough red peppers or cayenne in it so when 4 drops of this liquid are put in ½ cup of water it tastes strong.

Drinking an infusion made with mayweed upon going to bed, with a little ginger or cayenne, will cure a cold or throw off the first attack of fever, and if there are symptoms of the grippe, place a hot brick to the feet, with a cloth wet with vinegar, and wrapped in a dry flannel; drink freely of mayweed with cayenne; and in most cases it will effect a cure.

An infusion of the flowers of elder is a sovereign remedy and its action is increased when flowers are mixed with peppermint leaves.

Take equal parts of elder flowers, peppermint leaves and yarrow leaves, mix thoroughly. Use 1 teaspoon to each cup of water. Boil 4 or 5 minutes, strain and drink as hot as possible before retiring.

Use oil of peppermint freely, rubbing it on the forehead, in front and back of the ears and each side of the nose. Inhale through each nostril. If the throat is affected pour 3 or 4 drops in a dish of boiling hot water and inhale fumes. Soak the feet in hot water at bedtime and take a good sweat, if possible.

Remain in the house a few days, adopt a vegetable diet, and take warm demulcent drinks, such as flaxseed, mullein, and slippery elm, in order to excite a gentle sweat.

Take plenty of good physic with hot herbal teas.

Boil heaping teaspoon cumin seed to each cup of water for 5 or 6 minutes. Strain when cool and add honey to taste.

Mrs. R. C. D., 1950

A decoction made with dragon roots will cure the worst case of flu.

Black snakeroot is a sure cure for flu, colds and helps pneumonia. I have used it all my life and my mother used it before me. We are Cherokee Indians.

Mrs. M. C., 1949

The ground or beaten root of coral bean made into a tea is used with success for flu to clear the lungs and cool fever in parts of Louisiana where the bush was found.

Letter, 1923

Boil down, gently for 3 hours, a handful of angelica root, in about 1 quart of water: then, straining it off, add best virgin honey sufficient to make it into a balsam or syrup; and take 2 teaspoons every night and morning, as well as often in the day. If there be any hoarseness, or sore throat, add a few niter drops.

Other botanicals used for flu: august flowers [*Amphiachyris dracunculoides*], varieties of mountain mints [*Koellia*], horsemint [*Mo-*

narda punctata], bull nettle root [*Solanum carolinense*], balsam pear [*Momordica charantia*], etc.

ASIATIC FLU

At the first symptoms, clean the nostrils, dampen index finger and dip same in powdered lovage root; insert into nostrils, so they are dry. Repeat this 2 or 3 times a day. Recipe is harmless.

CONVALESCING AFTER FLU

Steep in 1 quart of whiskey ½ ounce each of Turkey rhubarb, Virginia snakeroot, golden seal root, wormwood herb, and Jamaica ginger and 2 grains of capsicum. Take tablespoon night and morning.

COUGH AFTER FLU

Ordinary grated horseradish, eaten at frequent intervals during the day and in connection with food at the table, if food is eaten at all, has been found remarkably efficacious in banishing the distressing cough that frequently lingers after all the other symptoms of the grippe have gone.

FROSTBITE

Use gentle friction in a warm room, using enough cold water or snow to prevent too rapid reaction and consequent pain in affected part.

Soak parts affected in kerosene oil.

Make a poultice of roasted turnips and bind them on parts frosted after turnips have been chilled.

Take the inner bark of elder, simmer it in hen's oil, and rub the affected part with it twice a day over a warm fire; at the same time wrap the frost bitten part in a piece of woollen cloth well greased with the same. In a few days this will effect a cure.

FROZEN FEET

Put enough boiling water in a pail to cover the feet; in this dissolve
all the powdered alum possible; as soon as you can bear it place
your feet in the water and soak them for 2 hours, adding hot water
and alum as the water in the pail cools, keeping it as hot as it
can be borne.

Mrs. M. W. Ellsworth, 1897

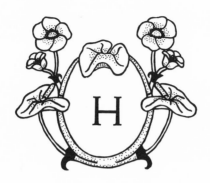

HAYFEVER

Rub the ears briskly when there is the slightest indication of fulness in the nose. Rub thoroughly until the ears are red and hot.

Inhale fumes of ground coffee sprinkled over hot coals.

Make a pillow of fresh hemlock boughs and lie on it and relief will follow and continue as long as the odor remains.

Take fresh horseradish roots, wash and grind, skin and all, in your kitchen meat grinder and fill a 1 quart fruit jar ½ full. Pour in white vinegar enough to barely cover the ground horseradish. Gas will form in the jar which must be tightly capped with the usual rubber gasket under the metal cap. When attacked by a fit of sneezing, remove the metal cap and place your nose deep into the jar, inhale deeply and be sure to replace the cap quickly to preserve the gas. Only freshly ground horseradish is of any use. Renew the entire mixture about every 5 days.

Mix 3 drops each of peppermint oil, oil of rosemary, oil of cloves and any other pungent oil; put in a tiny bottle and inhale occasionally to clear the head.

Take the fresh milkweed, crush it in a piece of cheese cloth and inhale it. The milkweed must be crushed fresh daily. Carry it in your pocket by putting a piece of heavy wax paper around it or place in a small jar—lay it on pillow at night and breathe, breathe and breathe.

Mrs. C. W. C., 1950

Take 2 cups of boiling water add 1 heaping teaspoon of wild plum bark and 1 level teaspoon each of coltsfoot and mullen herb. Allow to steep for 20 minutes. Drink wineglassful 2 or 3 times a day.

Old medical paper

The worst case of hayfever that ever existed can be immunized by the use of the leaves and flowers of common ragweed and goldenrod. Mix the herbs and use ½ ounce to each pint of boiling water. Steep 10 minutes. Strain. Take wineglassful 4 times daily.

HEADACHES

BILIOUS HEADACHE

Take ½ ounce rhubarb, 1 ounce carbonate of magnesia; mix intimately; keep well corked in glass bottle. Dose, 1 teaspoon, in milk and sugar, the first thing in the morning; repeat until cured.

Steep a pinch of senna leaves and chamomile flowers in a little boiling water. Strain and drink when cold.

Steep a pinch of senna leaves with a little sage and a dash of ginger in 1 cup of boiling water. Strain and drink when cool.

DISSIPATION, MENTAL EXHAUSTION OR MENSTRUAL PERIOD

Stir a teaspoon of powdered seeds of guarana in 1 cup of boiling water and drink while warm.

Drink a cup of clear coffee with the juice of a lemon.

Mrs. M. S.

NERVOUS HEADACHE

Drink a hot tea made with motherwort herb or dittany herb.

Make a strong decoction of hop tea and take a wineglassful every ½ hour or hour as desired or according to response.

Drink an infusion made of equal parts of wood betony, wood sage, and ground pine.

Brew a tea of equal parts of betony, marjoram, rosemary, and sage. Drink a wineglassful morning and night.

Boil 1 ounce of lady slipper root in a pint of water for 10 minutes. Strain and bottle liquid. Dose, a wineglassful when desired and as a sleep inducer on retiring.

Pour 2 pints of boiling water on ½ ounce of each of skullcap herb and chamomile flowers. Let it stand and cool. Strain and take wineglassful frequently.

Take teaspoon each of skullcap and valerian root. Steep in 1 cupful of boiling water. Strain when cool and drink. Another method: Take powdered botanicals with peppermint tea.

One quart of cider, 3 tablespoons of white mustard seed, 3 of burdock seed, a small horseradish root, well steeped together. To be kept in a bottle well corked; dose, a wineglassful 2 or 3 times a day.

Exercise on horseback, a cold bath every morning, an attention to the diet, and the bowels, together with the following infusion, will effect the cure; take scullcap, skunk cabbage root, lady slipper root, each, in coarse powder, a tablespoon; boiling water, a pint; mix; steep near hot fire for 1 or 2 hours, when cold, sweeten. The dose is a tablespoon every 2 hours.

J. King, M.D., 1855

SICK HEADACHE

The juice of a lime or small lemon in ½ glass of cold water, with a little baking soda stirred in. Drink it while it foams, at the time of getting up in the morning.

The juice of a lemon in a cup of hot water is excellent. Follow with a good laxative.

Take a shovelful of clean wood ashes; put them into clean cold water; when it has settled, drink the water: it may cause vomiting; if it does, the headache will be relieved the sooner.

A pinch of salt on the tongue, followed 10 minutes afterward by a drink of cold water.

Take a spoonful of finely powdered charcoal in a small glass of warm water. Charcoal absorbs the gases produced by the fermentation of undigested food.

Take a teaspoon of powdered charcoal in molasses every morning, and wash it down with a little tea; or, drink ½ glass of raw rum or gin, and drink freely of mayweed tea.

Dr. A. A. Benezet, 1826

Eat the meat of a peach stone. This has been tried in my mother's family since I was a child, and the remedy was never known to fail.

The Kansas Home Cook Book, 1879

Nothing is better than a cleaning-out of the stomach. To do this quickly and easily, simply drink lukewarm water until you can't drink any more. Drink until you are full to running over, and your stomach will empty itself without any difficult retching. Follow the cleaning out with a small dose of bicarbonate of soda in water, and lie down to rest.

Make a tea of mullein seeds and drink freely.

Whenever the symptoms are felt coming on, drink a cupful of boneset tea.

Gather sumach leaves in summer, and spread in the sun a few days to dry. Then powder them fine, and smoke morning and evening for 2 weeks, also whenever there are symptoms of approaching headache. Use a new clay pipe. If these directions are adhered to, this medicine will surely effect a permanent cure.

EXTERNAL APPLICATIONS

Nervous headaches will sometimes yield to a hot foot bath and hot water applications to the back of the neck.

Wet cloth in cold water, and lay it on the back of the neck. Fold a towel smoothly over it, and very often it will soothe the weary brain, and quiet the nerves better than an opiate.

Peel and slice raw potatoes and bind them on the forehead in a cloth that reaches around the head.

Stir baking soda in cold water, dampen a rag or towel and tie it around the head.

Wet cloth with spirits of camphor and sprinkle with black pepper. Apply to the head.

A ground mustard poultice, applied to the back of the neck, between the shoulders, is good.

The root of cow parsnip boiled in sweet oil and the head rubbed therewith, will cure headache and drowsiness, lethargy, etc.

The oil from anise scented goldenrod prepared in essence, and used to scent snuff with, is good for those persons who are constantly troubled with headache.

Cajeput oil applied to the temples or inhaled through the nostrils often cures violent headaches.

If those who are suffering from violent headache, bind fresh mint across their forehead, they will soon experience relief and ease.

Hop pillows are good for nervous patients and those afflicted with headaches and neuralgia. Heat them well and place under the head.

Fresh leaves of common burdock, fresh roots of poke, fresh garlic, garden onions, wild onions or mustard seed. Apply any one of the above to the soles of the feet.

John Monroe, *The American Botanist
and Family Physician,* 1824

The most excruciating head and toothache have often been suddenly dispelled by applying horseradish in fresh shavings or bruised garlic, between 2 fine pieces of muslin, to the bend of both arms, or the hams. Another simple remedy of equal efficacy, in periodical headaches, especially in the morning, is a thin piece of fresh lemon peel freed from the soft fibrous part, and placed on each of the temples, before the volatile oil be evaporated.

HICCUP or HICCOUGH

Place the hand flat upon the pit of the stomach, immediately below the cartilage forming the end of the breast bone, and making firm pressure. Should this prove unsuccessful, place a firm roll of muslin on the place, securing it by a bandage bound tightly around the body. In an hour this may be removed, and it will be found that the hiccough has entirely disappeared.

Mrs. M. Ellsworth, 1897

Thrust the tongue out of the mouth and hold it there for a short time.

Hold the breath as long as possible.

Drink as many successive swallows of water as possible without breathing.

Chew and swallow finely crushed ice.

Block the ears with a finger of each hand while taking 5 sips of water from a glass on a table.

Take about a teacupful of cold water in 9 sips.

Drink cold soda water.

Eating sugar, or drinking sugared water. The latter is often given to infants.

Hiccups in children are immediately stopped by giving them a lump of sugar saturated with wine vinegar. The same remedy was tried on adults with similarly instantaneous success.

Eat a little damson plum preserves or make a tea from the damson root.

Split a tomato, or a lemon, push in a lump of sugar and suck the piece through the sugar.

Take a teaspoon of sharp vinegar with a little essence of peppermint added.

Often a few mint leaves well chewed will relieve, or sip peppermint tea.

Put ¼ teaspoon of powdered cinchona bark in 2 ounces of peppermint tea, and give 1 teaspoon every 5 or 10 minutes until relieved.

Take 5 drops oil of amber in mint tea every 10 minutes until hiccup ceases.

Put as much dill seed, finely powdered, as will lie on a shilling into 2 spoonfuls of syrup of black cherries, and take it presently.

Chew a teaspoon of dill seed.

If hiccup is caused by flatulence or wind, drink a warm infusion of fennel seed. Another recipe advises chewing the seeds.

Take warm carminatives or cordials.

A camphor lozenge, or a little camphor in water, will stop a hiccup at once.

A single drop of oil of cinnamon on a bit of loaf sugar held in the mouth till dissolved, then gently swallowed, was said to be an infallible cure. Another recipe advises 3 drops of oil of cinnamon on a lump of sugar.

Take 1 ounce rhubarb, ¼ ounce cinnamon, bruised, ¼ ounce aniseed, bruised. Boil gently in 1 pint of water, for 1 hour; strain, sweeten with honey, and give ½ teaspoon when the symptoms are most troublesome.

HIVES or NETTLE RASH

Take ¼ teaspoon of baking soda in water each morning for 3 mornings then miss 3 mornings until 9 doses. Also take a warm bath with 1 pound of soda in the water. A sure relief.

Steep 1 teaspoon of ground ivy herb in 1 cup of boiling water. Drink a cupful of this tea each day for 3 days.

Drink freely of infusions made of red clover flowers, sassafras, catnip herb, or American brooklime.

Drink freely of a decoction made of ginseng roots.

Take 4 ounces of squills, 4 ounces of seneca snakeroot, pulverized fine, put in 8 pounds of water, boil down to 4 pounds; strain, and add 4 pounds of honey; boil down to 6 pounds. Add 1 grain of emetic tartar to each ounce, stir it warm, and it is fit for use. For a dose, take from 1 to 3 teaspoons.

Make an infusion with slippery elm with water. Use as a wash and drink the tea several times a day.

Drink freely of an infusion made with cheese plant.

EXTERNAL APPLICATIONS

Bathe hives with a strong solution of baking soda or with strong vinegar. Slightly diluted ammonia will relieve the intense itching. The same is true of alcohol, which may be used pure.

For children, add a teaspoon of vinegar to a cupful of water and bathe the parts affected.

Rub hives with buckwheat flour.

HYPOCHONDRIA

An infusion made of rosemary herb has long been used as a placebo for hypochondriacs. The tea has an aromatic medicinal taste and may be taken by teaspoonful or as needed.

One ounce each of aloes, gentian root, orange peel (not dyed), juniper berries, anise seed in 1 pint of gin. Let mixture stand 2 weeks and then strain. Dose, 1 tablespoon twice a day. In case of fainting, with a sensation of dying, motherwort tea, with a teaspoon of spirits of camphor, may be given.

HYSTERIA

The sudden effusion of water on the face and hands, while the fit is on, and especially immersing the feet in cold water, will afford relief.

Old English recipe

A hot foot bath, or warm bath is often useful.

Warm infusion of chamomile flowers in small and frequent doses is generally effective. The tea is especially useful for affections peculiar to nervous females.

Take a quantity of Canada or whiteroot [*Asclepias tuberosa*], and boil it in fair water; strain it, and boil the liquor down so thick that it may be made into pills. When the disorder is coming on, take 2 or 3 pills at a dose.

Take the leaves of motherwort and thoroughwort, and poplar bark, from the root of the tree. Pound these fine, and sift them through a fine sieve. Mix with molasses, and make it into pills, and take 4 of them when the disorder is coming on. This will settle the head, and make every thing as calm as a clock.

P. F. Bowker, 1836

A tea of boneset, green wheat, or motherwort usually affords relief. When the nerves are much agitated, a dose or 2 of lady slipper root has a good effect. Costiveness should be obviated by cathartics.

Dr. D. Rogers, 1824

Two teaspoons of the powdered root of skunk cabbage in spirits and water procured immediate relief in one of the most violent hysteric cases I ever met with. On repeating the trials with the same patient, it afforded more lasting benefit than any other medicine.

Elias Smith, Physician, 1826

The following mixture will be found useful in severe cases: skunk cabbage root ½ ounce; skullcap herb ½ ounce; lady slipper ½ ounce; lobelia ½ ounce; capsicum 2 drachms, alcohol 1 pint; compound spirits of lavender 1 pint; ether and ammonia, each 4 ounces. Mix, and let stand 2 weeks, frequently shaking it. Dose, 1 or 2 teaspoons, as often as required.

H. R. Stout, M.D., 1886

When traced to impaired natural action: Take equal portions of pennyroyal and wormwood, steep in boiling water, simmer until virtues of the herbs are extracted. It should then be allowed to cool, and ½ pint be taken twice or thrice a day, succeeded on each occasion by a compound asafoetida pill, until the desired relief is afforded.

ALLEGED PREVENTIVES

Take caraway seeds, finely pounded, with a small portion of ginger and salt, spread upon bread and butter, and eat every day, especially early in the morning and at night before going to bed.

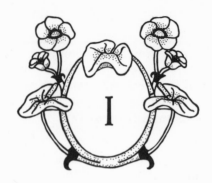

INSOMNIA

The usual cause of this trouble is too much blood in the brain, and those thus affected will often find it advantageous to raise the head of the bed a foot higher, and then sleep on a thick hair pillow so as to bring the head a little higher than the shoulders. The object of this is to make the work of the heart harder in throwing blood to the brain. Sometimes rising for a time, wrapping up and sitting in a chair with the feet, if possible, at the fire. Take a short nap in this manner, and then return to bed. After continued mental labor, a light lunch before retiring will often induce sleep, as the work of digestion draws the blood from the brain to the stomach. Or have the room dimly lighted, lie with head propped up. Select some object a little to one side. Look steadily at this. Let the eyes get well a-weary, and refreshing sleep will soon follow.

Miss M. C. Cooke, 1889

A hearty meal just before retiring, and a seat near fire after a long, cold walk will usually cause a deep sleep.

Wet a cloth in cold water; and lay it on the back of the neck. Fold a towel smoothly over it, and very often it will soothe the weary brain, and quiet the nerves better than an opiate.

Hot water used both internally and externally is highly recommended as a cure for insomnia. Bathing the feet in hot water is said to be particularly good.

Nervous persons are often troubled with wakefulness, caused by a tendency of blood to the brain. Rubbing the body and extremities with a brush, towel, or the hands will promote circulation and withdraw the blood from the brain. A cold bath often has the same effect.

A mustard foot bath is often beneficial.

Take a cup of hot milk, nicely sweetened and flavored with freshly grated nutmeg, the last thing at night. One should take care that the feet are comfortably warm.

Half teaspoon nutmeg gratings and a pinch of red pepper in ½ tumbler of hot milk in which 2 teaspoons of honey have been dissolved.

Eat a dish of baked onions or try eating a thin slice of bread and butter, sprinkled with a little cayenne pepper. This is sure to induce sleep, but do not try the remedy too often, for the pepper would soon injure the stomach if too frequently used.

Take a teaspoon of lime flowers to a teacup of boiling water. Strain while still warm, add a few gratings of nutmeg.

Try drinking a large cupful of hot lemonade or hot ginger tea just before retiring.

Infuse cowslip flowers as you would if making tea. Let it stand 5 minutes. Milk can be added. Drink at bed time.

Make a mild tea of Jerusalem oak herb, and drink it warm, as you would any other tea, before going to bed.

J. Marquart, 1867

The juice of lettuce mixed with oil of roses, and applied to the forehead, is good to produce sleep and ease the headache.

A harmless and certain soporific, especially useful in nervous headache was made by steeping heaping teaspoon of *Passiflora incarnata* in a cupful of boiling water and allowing it to steep 7 or 8 minutes. Strain and drink while warm.

Wash the head in a decoction of dill seeds and smell of it frequently.

A pillow made with hops is sometimes used for sleeplessness. To prepare it, fill a small pillow case with hops, which have been sprinkled with alcohol, to bring out the active principle. Also drink a cup of warm tea made with hops before retiring.

Take 1 ounce each of scullcap herb, hops, blue vervain herb, chamomile, and ½ ounce of valerian root. Mix thoroughly. Place a teaspoon of the mixture in a cup, and over them pour ½ teacupful of boiling water. Infuse 10 minutes and drink warm on retiring.

Valerian root serves to quiet nerves, prevent spasms and procure easy sleep, without stupefying. When a person cannot sleep, put a teaspoon of the powdered root into a teacupful of strong pennyroyal tea, warm enough to drink, and take it when in bed at night and it causes an easy refreshing sleep.

Elias Smith, Physician, 1826

Lady slipper root was a very popular sedative in domestic practice. The powdered root was taken in teaspoonful doses in sugar water or herbal tea such as chamomile or linden flowers. An excellent tea is also made by mixing equal parts of lady slipper root with scullcap herb. Allow 1 teaspoon of mixture to steep in boiling water for 6 or 7 minutes. Strain and drink warm before retiring.

RECIPES FOR INFANTS AND CHILDREN

Garlic applied to the feet of children quiets and produces sleep.

P. E. Sanborn, 1836

For infants, make an infusion of burdock seeds. Give warm tea slightly sweetened. A warm infusion of catnip was very popular in domestic practice.

For nightmare in children or adults give warm tea made of chamomile flowers.

Nightmare in infants and children. A whiff of cologne is generally enough to bring the sufferer back to its ordinary world.

Miss T. S. Shute, 1878

INTOXICATION

To remove the effects produced by an excess of wine, etc., drink a wineglassful of olive oil. It will prevent the hurtful fumes from rising. It will have the same effect if taken before an intended debauch.

When a person begins to feel the effects of liquor, eat 6 or 8 lumps of loaf sugar, and its beneficial results will be felt immediately.

Tartar emetic, 8 grains; rosewater, 4 ounces. Mix. Put a tablespoon into the whole quantity of liquor drunk each day by the patient, and let him take it as usual. Be careful not to exceed a tablespoon or ½ ounce.

The American Family Receipt Book, 1854

To cure the fit of drunkenness, take ½ ounce of mindererus spirit in a cupful of water. Repeat dose every 15 minutes.

A man who is helplessly intoxicated may almost immediately restore the faculties and powers of locomotion by taking ½ teaspoon of chloride of ammonium in a goblet of water. A wineglassful of strong vinegar will have the same effect and is frequently resorted to by drunken soldiers.

A cold infusion of boneset has speedily restored the tone of the stomach after drunkenness.

C. S. Rafinesque, 1828

A decoction made with golden seal root with a little capsicum and forced nutrition was a remedy to help overcome chronic alcoholism.

Take ½ ounce each of sassafras, sarsaparilla and burdock root, boil in 1 quart of water until reduced to 1 pint. Drink this instead of water, tea or coffee. It will kill the want of liquor.

The following was believed to cure the cravings of the worst drunkard in the land: Take 1 pound of best, fresh, quill red Peruvian bark, powdered, and soak it in 1 pint of diluted alcohol. Afterward strain and evaporate it down to ½ pint. Dose, a teaspoon every 3 hours the first and 2nd day, and occasionally moisten the tongue between doses. It acts like quinine, and the patient can tell by a headache if he is getting too much. The 3rd day take as previous, but reduce the dose to ½ teaspoon. Afterward reduce the dose to 15 drops, and then down to 10, then down to 5 drops. To make a cure it takes from 5 to 15 days, and in extreme cases 30 days. Seven days are about the average in which a cure can be effected.

The Modern Home Cook Book
and Family Physician, about 1880

ITCH

Lemon juice rubbed on the inflamed part is recommended, and we have known a sliced onion dipped in salt to have that effect, but the latter makes the skin very tender.

Apply a little mutton tallow to area of itch.

Apply a paste made with oatmeal and oil of bay.

Barber's itch or scabies: flour of sulphur with enough glycerin to make an ointment. Use hog's lard instead of glycerin for salve.

The best specific is an ointment composed of 2 ounces flowers of sulphur, 2 drachms carbonate of potash, 4 ounces lard; to be well rubbed in, night and morning.

Take ½ pound hog's lard, 4 ounces spirits of turpentine, 2 ounces flour-sulphur, and mix them together cold; apply it to the ankles, knees, wrists, and elbows, and rub it on the palms of the hands; if there be any raw spots, apply a little 3 nights when going to bed.

Two tablespoons lard, 1 of black pepper, 1 of ground mustard; boil all together, and when taken off and nearly cold add 1 tablespoon flour of sulphur. Anoint with this 3 evenings successively just before going to bed. Do not change bed clothes or wearing clothes during the time. After this, wash with castile soap suds, and change all the clothing that has been worn or touched.

To 3 ounces fresh unsalted butter add a lump of beeswax the size of a hickory nut, 5 tablespoons ground juniper berries and 3 tablespoons ground cloves. Melt and mix well and when nearly cool add 1 tablespoon sulphur.

Boil elecampane roots in vinegar, mix with fresh lard, beating thoroughly.

The fresh juice or a strong decoction of dried root of elecampane is useful as a wash for itch.

Elliot states that the negroes of Carolina use the leaves of *Kalmia angustifolia* and *Kalmia hirsuta* in a strong wash to cure the itch of men and dogs; it smarts, but cures effectually.

C. S. Rafinesque, 1830

Laurel leaves stewed in lard, make an excellent ointment for scald head or itch.

The burs of sweet fern, when pounded and made into an ointment, are most sure to cure that inveterate disorder, commonly called the itch. It can also be made into an ointment, and used with good success for salt rheum. When the burs cannot be had, use the bush and the buds.

The powdered root of poke, mixed with a little lard, is a good ointment for itch, scald head and the like.

Take 2 teaspoons yellow dock root, 6 teaspoons poke root, 1 teaspoon hog lard. Mix in 1 pint of water—boil down to ½ pint. Apply night and morning.

The juice, decoction, or ointment of the root of the narrow dock is a certain remedy for the itch, if persevered in. We are also informed by good authority, that the leaves are equally as good as the roots, and may be used by bruising and then rubbing them upon the affected parts. The broad leaved dock, it is likewise said, proves equally efficacious with the narrow kind.

An itch ointment is also made in the Southern States by melting sweet gum with sweet oil or lard, and is said to be very useful.

INTERNAL MEDICINE FOR ITCH

In 1 pint of gin steep of black cherry bark, prickly ash, and yellow dock root, each 1 ounce, adding ½ pint of water; and drink 2 glasses a day.

Make a syrup of the juice of sorrel and fumitory. This is a sovereign remedy for that troublesome disorder. Use it inwardly, and the juice of sorrel and vinegar, as a wash, outwardly.

JAUNDICE

Take the yolk of a hen's egg, a teaspoon of lemon juice, a teaspoon of sugar; mix; take this 3 mornings, and then miss 3; repeat it if necessary.

Take whites of 2 eggs, beat them up well in a gill of water; take this, a little every morning, it will soon do good.

Take a tablespoon of lemon juice several times a day.

Drink all the new cider [before it ferments] you can.

Take 2 oranges, and pare them very thin; then chop the peel as fine as suet, to which put 2 quarts of cold water, and simmer them till reduced to a pint and a ½; strain and bottle it. Of this mixture take, for 3 successive mornings, ½ a pint, which will perfectly cure the patient of jaundice.

Eat dandelion greens as often as possible.

A decoction of dandelion root will correct an unhealthy state of the stomach and liver. It is diuretic and very beneficial in jaundice.

As the stomach is usually disordered, it is well to give an emetic, and after it has acted freely administer a gentle purge. Should there be a coldness about the feet or body use the hot bath, or bathe the whole body with hot vinegar and water. A decoction made of dandelion root and barberry root may be drunk freely. If these do not give immediate relief, take the following: golden seal root and capsicum, of each, 1 dram; bitter root, and white poplar, of each, 2 drams. Cover with boiling water. When cool, add ½ pint gin. Dose, a wineglassful 3 times a day.

An emetic, followed by a cathartic, should be given once every week, and in the meantime take the following: of white poplar, prickly ash bark, wild cherry bark, golden seal, each, in coarse powder, a handful; horseradish root, mustard seed, each in coarse powder, ½ handful; good cider 1 gallon. Mix; steep near a fire for 24 hours. Dose, ½ gill 3 or 4 times a day.

Boil 1 pound wild cherry bark in 1 quart water till reduced to 1 pint. Sweeten and add a little rum to preserve, or if to be used immediately, omit the rum. Dose, 1 small wineglassful 3 times a day, on an empty stomach. Give ½ doses to children.

Take of wild cherry bark, 2 ounces, bloodroot and goldthread root, ½ ounce; put into a pint of brandy. Dose, from a teaspoon to a tablespoon, morning and night.

Take daily ½ pint of strong tea made of peach tree leaves.

Take inner bark of a peach tree; make a strong tea and give a teaspoon before each meal for 5 days, then stop 5 days and repeat if not cured.

Drink 2 cupfuls of tea made of boneset herb, every day for a week or two. No other medicine need be taken at the time this is used.

Boil 1 ounce barberry bark in 1 pint of water for 20 minutes. Squeeze out the bark and strain the liquor. Dose, 1 tablespoon 3 or 4 times a day.

A tea made from oats is good.

A gill of the ashes of the bark of walnut steeped in cider, and a gill of liquor drunk in the morning, fasting, is good.

Take a large handful of black alder; cut it up fine and boil it in a quart of old cider. Let it cool, and then drink of it freely. This is very good to remove jaundice.

Take the juice of cinquefoil or five-fingered grass, in new milk, every morning before eating or drinking, in the following manner. To every gill of milk add 1 glass of the juice; this must be drunk while warm; continue this treatment for a number of days, and your complexion will satisfy you of its good effects. For what you see with your own eyes, you will be sure there is no deception in.

P. F. Bowker, 1836

Make a syrup of the juice of hops and sugar in the following manner: Pound the hops, and press out the juice, then add the same quantity of loaf sugar you have of juice, and simmer whole as long as any scum rises. If the weather be warm, a little brandy is necessary to prevent souring. It is perfectly safe, and may be used at discretion. The best time to take it is in the morning, on an empty stomach.

Take ½ pint of the last milk that can be obtained from a cow, and a small handful of yellow blowed celandine; put into a cloth and pound them; then squeeze it till the juice is out, and then mix and drink the whole, while warm, every morning before eating, for the space of 9 mornings in succession, which will generally be sufficient; but if obstinate, or of long standing, it will be necessary to omit it for 9 mornings, and then take it for the same space as before, which will be sufficient to cure the disorder in its worst form and longest standing.

KIDNEYS

TO PROMOTE URINE

Sit over the steam of warm water. Or, drink largely of a decoction of turnips, sweetened with clarified honey. Or, drink of warm lemonade.

The juice of artichokes, mixed with an equal quantity of white wine, powerfully promotes urine.

The seeds of cucumbers are good to provoke urine and cleanse the urinary passages.

Take a tablespoon of French brandy in milk just from the cow every morning.

Dr. B. W. James, 1852

An elderly lady whose kidneys ceased functioning was fed the soft coconut jelly of the unripe fruit. Kidneys were restored to normal discharge.

The bark of the root of gooseberry bush being steeped strong, is one of the best things known for strangury.

The common mulberry bush, made into a tea, and drunk freely, is good for all urinary obstructions. It is perfectly harmless in its operation.

The fresh roots of white hellebore, pulverized, and applied to the bowels, promote the discharge of urine.

White hellebore is a powerful emetic; and so poisonous that if eaten by swine or fowls, it proves immediately mortal.

J. Monroe, 1824

Steep the roots of asparagus in cold water, after being well bruised, or split into shreds, and let the patient drink of the water often through the course of the day. It will increase the discharge of urine in a short time, and relieve strangury.

H. Howard, 1857

Take good ripe pumpkin seeds, dry them and pound as well as you can conveniently; add 1 quart of good gin to 1 gill of the pounded seeds. Keep it in some warm place till the gin is tolerably well tinctured with the seeds. Drink a wineglass of this 3 times a day before eating. This will be found to answer your most sanguine expectations.

P. F. Bowker, 1836

Failure of the baby to make water: If the baby should not pass its water for a day or 2 following its birth, no apprehensions need be felt. But if a longer time should elapse, it may be well to administer to it a little watermelon seed, pumpkin seed, or flaxseed tea, either of which will probably produce the desired effect.

Mrs. E. B. Duffey, 1882

Drink freely of a tea made of pumpkin seed, watermelon seed, queen-of-the-meadow root, marshmallow root, etc. At the same time apply warm fomentations over the region of the bladder, as stramonium leaves; hops and lobelia herb; lobelia and sassafras leaves; pounded onions or garlic.

J. King, M.D., 1864

The watery extract of juniper berries is good for suppression of urine in old age.

After 20 years of suffering, I have been cured of bladder trouble by drinking an infusion made with juniper berries.

F. M., 1953

An infusion of the leaves of buchu is good for increasing the secretion of urine and removing obstructions in the bladder. Old people especially will find great benefit by taking the following preparation: Pour 1 pint of water upon 1 ounce of buchu leaves and simmer gently for 1 hour, strain, and take a wineglassful 3 times per day.

Mrs. A. Matteson, 1894

Take 2 ounces buchu leaves; 2 ounces uva ursi; 1 ounce juniper berries; pulverize and mix well. Dose, 1 teaspoon in a cup of boiling water, steep 4 or 5 minutes; strain and drink.

Letter, 1931

Buckthorn berries steeped in water, to make a strong tea. Take a wineglassful 2 or 3 times a day.

Knotgrass is very useful for strangury, provoking urine and easing pains in the bladder.

An infusion of silver grass was used in Florida, where the plant is found, for bladder and kidney troubles.

C. Rye, 1935

Boil 1 ounce parsley piert herb for a few minutes in 1 pint of water. When cool strain. Dose 1 wineglassful twice a day.

Gipsy recipe

A decoction of horsetail grass or leaves of sheepberry is drunk as a remedy for dysurea. It is said to be quick in effect. Used by the Chippewa Indians.

The kidney root in the form of strong tea, made by boiling the root, increases the discharge by urine, and strengthens the urinary organs. It is useful in suppression of urine, bloody urine, gravel, and weakness of these parts generally.

W. M. Hand, 1820

Drink freely of tea made of cleavers. Best made by steeping the herb overnight in cold water.

Mullein leaves are good steeped with strawberry leaves and clivers in water, for kidney complaints, and obstructions of the urine.

Make a strong tea of clivers, mullein and the inner bark of witch hazel. Sweeten it with loaf sugar, and add a tablespoon of gin to every pint of tea. This is sure to give relief by carrying the disorder off in the water.

Drink freely of an infusion made with button weed.

Take ⅓ or ¼ piece of the leaf of *Bryophyllum pinnatum,* pour boiling water over it and allow to stand for several minutes. Drink this in place of water, 3 or more times a day.

Make an infusion of prickly pear cactus. Drink as needed.

TOO FREE, OR NO CONTROL OF URINE

When this affection is not a symptom of another disease, or debility in the system, such as stone in the bladder, palsy, etc., it can easily be cured. Take 1 ounce each of bistort root, white pond lily root, sumach berries, white poplar bark and 2 ounces rock candy. Bruise the roots and berries, and put down in 3 pints of water; simmer gently down to 1 quart. Pour this on 1 ounce of beth root powder; strain when cold, and take a wineglassful 3 times a day. The patient should be rubbed across the loins every morning with salt and water. Let the patient become accustomed to sleep either on side or face downwards.

Make a decoction of equal parts of wild cherry bark, hemlock bark and bayberry bark. Add a sufficient quantity of water to make a strong tea or decoction. While the patient is taking this decoction, let him take 15 or 20 drops of the balsam of copaiva in a tumbler of beth root tea 3 times a day. Diet should consist of boiled milk, and wheat flour, with a little nutmeg and cinnamon sprinkled on it. Avoid tea, coffee and as little as possible other liquids.

Take 2 ounces of Peruvian bark; steep it in 1 quart of wine 24 hours; add drachm of alum. Dose, from a spoonful to a wineglassful 2 or 3 times a day.

Simmer 2 ounces of Peruvian bark in 3 pints of water down to 1 quart. Take ½ wineglassful 3 or 4 times per day.

An infusion of yarrow herb will relieve those who can not retain their water.

Take mullein or catnip tea; or both mixed.

A plaster of the tormentil root and vinegar is good. It should be externally applied to the back against the kidneys.

CHRONIC KIDNEY COMPLAINT

Take 1 ounce each of the following: dandelion root, burdock root, bittersweet, gentian root, wild cherry bark, horehound herb, pipsissewa, buchu leaves, yellow dock root, snake root, juniper berries, columbo root; 2 ounces sarsaparilla root and ½ ounce pleurisy root. Mix the botanicals together then add 3 quarts of boiling water. Then set the preparation on the stove in a proper vessel and let it boil slow (well covered) down to 2 quarts. Strain while warm and add 1 pound of sugar. Shake it well and set it in a cool place for use. Dose, from 1 to 2 teaspoons 3 times a day ½ hour before eating.

Dr. D. Winter, 1856

SCALDING URINE, OR IRRITATION IN ABSENCE OF SYSTEMIC OR ORGANIC DISEASE

This may be readily relieved by using freely of a tea of marshmallow root, or spearmint, thimbleberry leaves, black raspberry, watermelon seed, pumpkin seed, cleavers, whortleberry leaves, queen-of-the-meadow root, black currant root, etc. One or more of these may be combined together in form of tea, and sweetened with sugar or honey, as it best agrees with the patient.

Take 1 ounce buchu leaves; 1 ounce marshmallow root; ½ ounce couch grass root. Put mixture in 3 pints of water, bring to a boil and simmer for 15 minutes then strain. Dose, ½ teacupful warm every 2 hours during the day, and gradually reduce the dose to 3 times daily.

Nephritic plant is highly esteemed by some practitioners as a remedy in diseases of the urinary organs. The root may be sliced, infused in cold water, and drunk in moderate quantities, for suppressions of the urine, and especially when a painful scalding or burning sensation attends its discharge, or when it is voided by drops or in very small quantities.

H. Howard, 1857

A decoction made of slippery elm bark is most soothing for scalding urine. The decoction may be taken freely or as needed.

The most striking quality of the fleabane is its diuretic power, for which purpose it has been used for a long time in domestic practice, and has proved highly successful in many cases in the hands of regular practitioners. Steep heaping teaspoon of the dried herb in a cup of boiling water. Strain when cool. Drink cupful 2 or 3 times a day between meals.

R. E. Griffith, M.D., 1847

INFLAMMATION. PALLIATIVES FOR NEPHRITIC PAROXYSMS

Produce profuse sweating as soon as possible. Should the bowels be costive, a cathartic must be given. To relieve the pain in the kidneys, apply fomentations upon the back, just over the affected organ, renewing it as often as may be necessary. And to aid in urinating, and at the same time lessen the inflammation, the patient may drink freely of a cold tea of cleavers, or of pumpkin seeds, watermelon seeds, marshmallow root, elder blows, wild carrot herb, flowers and seeds, string bean pods, etc. Use considerable care during convalescence, to avoid cold, and overloading the stomach.

J. King, M.D., 1864

Drink the infusion made with dry pods of the common white soup bean or corn bean. When this is not readily obtained, the pods of the snap short bean will answer, and even the lima bean, though the latter is of inferior strength. Take a double handful of the pods to 3 quarts of water; boil slowly for 3 hours until it is reduced to 3 pints. Use no drink of any kind but this, the patient drinking as much as he conveniently can; it may be taken either hot or cold.

*The Modern Home Cook Book
and Family Physician,* about 1880

The bowels should be opened with Epsom salts, or jalap, and cream of tartar, and copious injections [enema] of warm water, or decoctions of emollient herbs. Injections are particularly appropriate in this disease, affording great relief as a local bath, besides aiding in procuring evacuations from the bowels, and they should never be omitted. The drinks should be warm flaxseed, slippery elm, balm tea, and gum-water, to which may be added a little cream of tartar.

G. Capron, M.D., and D. B. Slack, M.D., 1848

Give a steam bath, take cayenne and prickly ash, equal parts, make a strong decoction, and lay cloths wrung out over the parts affected, as hot as can be borne, and then a dry flannel outside of that, then prepare the following tea: One ounce each of tansy herb, dandelion roots, uva ursi, marshmallow roots, burdock seeds. Add 2 quarts of water, boil down to 1 quart; strain, add 1 teaspoon of ginger and sweeten with molasses. Give a wineglassful every hour for the first 4 hours; then give every 2 hours. Wash the patient down in tepid water, vinegar and cayenne, followed by friction over the parts affected. Let the food be light, and drink flaxseed or slippery elm tea. Keep the bowels moderately open with senna and ginger.

Mrs. A. Matteson, 1894

Catarrhal inflammation of kidneys was cured by the use of infusion made of spikenard root. A piece of the root 4 inches long, and as large as the little finger makes a pint or more, and should be drunk freely.

Take 5 to 10 grains of bearberry leaves—larger quantity is more effectual, and is readily borne by the stomach. The decoction may be made from ½ ounce of the leaves boiled for 10 minutes in a pint of water. From a wineglass to a gill of this may be taken every hour.

J. Bigelow, 1817

Drink freely of an infusion made of buchu leaves. Steep tablespoon of the leaves in a cup of boiling water. Strain when cool. Keep saucer over cup while steeping.

Boil 1 ounce of couch grass in 1½ pints of water for 5 minutes. Strain when cool. Dose, a wineglassful 5 or 6 times a day if possible.

Steep 1 ounce of slippery elm bark in 1 pint of boiling water for 2 hours in a closed vessel, then strain. Use freely as a drink for inflammatory diseases of kidneys or bowels.

Make a strong tea of cornsilk by steeping slowly in boiling water. Take wineglassful 3 or 4 times a day.

Take 4 drops of oil of sandalwood in a little water 3 times a day. As you urinate more freely reduce the dose.

A decoction of the marshmallows should be drunk constantly; it is a sovereign remedy in diseases of the urinary organs, and may be relied upon, as a specific in this.

Drink freely of a strong decoction made of burdock seeds.

An infusion of peach tree leaves taken several times a day or as required will cure bladder inflammation when other medicines have failed.

Mrs. B. R., 1951

Steep ½ ounce of the root of Joe-Pye-weed in 1 quart of rapidly boiling water. Cover and let set till well brewed. Drink a glassful every hour till all is used. After the first day drink 1 glassful a day. Patient will also get relief from that terrible pressure by sitting in a tub of very hot water.

Mrs. C. C., 1951

PUS IN URINE

Drink freely of infusions made with couch grass root.

Take a little more than a pint of water and a large pinch of kidney-wort and horsetail grass. Let stand in covered container overnight. In the morning strain and drink ½ glassful 4 times a day. The patient will have to discontinue eating meat, eggs, cheese and nuts with starches at the same meal. Avoid anything made with white flour.

BLOOD IN URINE

Drink infusion made with a teaspoon of horsetail grass steeped in boiling water for 5 minutes and strained.

Shepherd's purse herb is an excellent remedy for those persons who have blood mixed with their water as it passes from them.

A patient was suffering from severe bladder trouble with hemorrhages. The doctor took peach tree leaves, made a tea and let the patient drink it. It stopped the hemorrhage.

Mrs. C. E. Bigelow, Nurse, 1917

I lately attended one case of this kind [blood in the urine], which I cured by a strong decoction of peach tree leaves.

Dr. W. Beach, *The American Practice of Medicine*, 1833

In case the leaves of peach tree cannot be procured the bark may be used. When there is reason to suspect that the complaint proceeds from a stone lodged in the kidney, ureter, or bladder, the patient ought to drink freely of some mucilaginous drink, such as thick barley water, a tea of marshmallows, or elm bark, any or all of which may be sweetened with honey. Injections of the same may also be administered.

H. Howard, *An Improved System of Domestic Medicine,* 1857

Drink from a pint to a quart daily of decoction made from all parts of the plants high mallow or low mallow. A decoction of mullein leaves and horse-mint is also very good. A little horse-mint or spearmint may be added to the marshmallow decoction.

J. C. Gunn, M.D., 1862

GRAVEL AND STONES. ATTEMPTED TREATMENTS

Eating fresh strawberries was believed to prevent formation of stones.

Take a handful of common beans, or bean pods, dried and powdered; add 1 pint of cold water; let it stand 3 or 4 hours, and drink freely.

Make of bean leaves a strong tea, and drink freely.

Boil ½ pound of parsnips in a quart of water. Drink a glass of this morning and evening, and use no other drinks all the day. It usually cures in 6 weeks.

Take morning and evening a teaspoon of onions, calcined in a fire-shovel into white ashes, in white wine. An ounce will often dissolve the stone.

Let the patient drink a gill of red onion juice, and a pint of horse-mint tea, twice a day, morning and evening, but not together. The effect will be perceivable within 3 days. Reported to me by a man who says it will dissolve the stone.

The foregoing was communicated by a slave, to a Baptist minister of Virginia, who was cured by it, and afterwards bought the slave and set him free.

H. Howard, 1857

Take red onions and pound them, press out the juice, add an equal quantity of horse-mint herb juice, a tablespoon of each, well mixed together, to be taken 3 times a day before eating, and drink a strong tea of clivers and witch hazel bark.

Take of the tops, twigs, and roots of honeysuckle or gravel weed 2 ounces; milkweed root 1 ounce; horse-mint 1 ounce, boiling water 1 quart. Mix; steep near a fire in a covered vessel for 10 or 12 hours, then sweeten, and drink freely.

Boil 1 ounce clivers or cleavers in 1½ pints of water for 10 minutes. Strain and boil the liquid up again for 1 minute. Dose, a wineglassful twice daily, morning and night.

Take of cleavers 3 or 4 handfuls, cold rain or soft water 1 quart. Let it stand a couple of hours, and drink freely of it.

Boil ½ ounce of bearberry leaves in a pint of water 5 minutes. Strain when cool. Drink wineglassful 3 times a day.

A tea made of mountain mint has been found very effectual to relieve gravel, and that when other medicines had proved ineffectual. It is generally speaking, a fine, safe, diuretic and perspirative medicine.

Take of the fresh root of nephritic plant 1 ounce, cut it up in slices, pour 1 pint of cold water on it, let it stand 2 hours, and drink ½ gill repeating it 3 or 4 times a day.

Spleenwort allays the pain in the urinary passages, and gently carries off sand and gravel. Drink the infusion as a tea.

J. Monroe, 1824

A tea made of the seeds of wild carrot, and taken freely without any other diluting liquid, gives much relief to those who are afflicted with the gravel and stone.

Caution. Wild carrot bears a considerable resemblance to the muskrat root, which proves a fatal poison, if taken in any considerable quantity.

Take wild carrot root or seeds; queen-of-the-meadow root, garden parsley root; thimble-weed, each in coarse powder 1 ounce; boiling water 1½ pints; mix, and let it steep, in a covered vessel, near a fire for 24 hours, and then sweeten with sugar or honey. Dose, ½ gill 3 or 4 times a day.

J. King, M.D., 1864

Queen-of-the-meadow is a most valuable medicine for all obstructions of the urinary organs. Bad cases of gravel and dropsy have yielded to this plant alone. The dose is a teaspoon of the powdered root in a cupful of water 3 or 4 times per day, as the case may require. A decoction may be used instead of the powder. Boil 1 ounce of the cut root in 1½ pints of water for 20 minutes. Strain and bottle. Dose, a small wineglassful taken frequently 5 or 6 times a day.

A cupful of shave grass taken from time to time (not daily) eases the pains caused by gravel and stone disease, and above all relieves the sufferers who have difficulty in discharging their urine. For this it stands alone, is not to be replaced, and is invaluable.

Broom tops combined with queen-of-the-meadow and smartweed in equal parts effectually cures gravel and stone in the bladder.

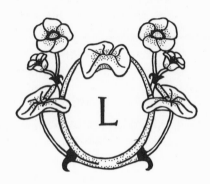

LEUCORRHEA

Also see FEMALE WEAKNESS.

Oregon grape root cures in 10 days according to an old record. It was discovered by the Kootenai Indians in the northwest where the shrub is found. Of their women, it may almost be said that they never have the disease—they cure it so promptly. Any woman thus afflicted can cure herself, even if she has had it for years. As a blood purifier, it is far superior to all so-called spring medicines. Boil ½ ounce of Oregon grape roots in 1 quart of water for 10 minutes. Strain when cool. Take a wineglassful 3 times a day.

Drink freely of the tea made of leaves and flowers of meadow sweet [*Spiraea tomentosa*] every day till cured. A certain safe and sure cure.

Dr. I. Richey, 1852

Steep 1 teaspoon of red alder bark in 1 cup of boiling water and allow to stand until cool. Drink 1 or 2 cups a day as needed.

A. Lewis, 1956

Make a strong syrup of yarrow herb, and take from 1 tablespoon to ⅔ of a wineglassful, 3 times a day.

Take 2 ounces of yarrow tops, 2 ounces of rose willow, 1 ounce garden parsley, and 4 ounces of burdock root. Boil in 4 quarts of water and 1 of new milk. Add sugar, and take a gill 3 times a day.

Take 2 parts powdered pleurisy root, 1 part powdered star root, mix and add enough oil of cinnamon to give a pleasant aromatic flavor. Give a teaspoon in a little cold water, on an empty stomach 3 times a day every day. This has been used in 25 cases with entire success.

Dr. B. W. James, 1852

DOUCHES

Use a strong decoction of common tea as a douche twice daily.

Use 2 tablespoons white vingar in 2 quarts of warm water.

Use 1 tablespoon witch hazel to 2 quarts of warm water.

Boil 3 teaspoons of cut white oak bark in a pint of water for 5 or 6 minutes. Strain and add the decoction to 1½ quarts of water. Use full quantity of the douche each morning. It seldom fails.

A decoction made from the roots of wild indigo is good as an injection in fetid leucorrhea, and wherever an antiseptic, cleansing and healing remedy is needed.

Use as douche night and morning, a decoction made with bistort, beth root or cranesbill. Also take at morning and night 1 wineglassful of the following decoction. To 3 pints of water add 2 ounces white pond lily root; 2 ounces unicorn root; 1 ounce wahoo root; 1 ounce golden seal root; and 1 ounce cinnamon. Simmer to 1 quart. Strain, pour boiling hot upon 1 ounce of grated nutmeg, ½ ounce ginger, ½ pound granulated sugar.

When the vaginal passage is very tender and irritated, an infusion of slippery elm bark is very soothing and may be used freely.

LIGHTNING

Application of cold water effects immediate relief from shock suffered from lightning.

Shower with cold water for 2 hours; if the patient does not show signs of life, put salt in the water, and continue to shower an hour longer.

A stroke of lightning, even though it may not kill, will invariably seriously derange the nervous system. In such cases it is essential that the animal warmth be maintained, which in consequence of the shock is liable to become diminished. If the respiration is feeble, artificial respiration may be employed, just as in the case of drowning; a little stimulant may also be administered, and mustard poultices applied across the region of the stomach and heart and also to the spine.

Stunned by thunder: Let a person of good strong lungs apply his mouth to the sufferer's holding at the same time his nostrils close, and blow his breath (as we say) as hard as he can into the sufferer's lungs; he must then leave him to expire while he gets his own breath, and then repeat the effort as soon and as often as he can, perhaps a hundred times, if self respiration does not take place sooner. A reed or pipe like a weaver's quill may be made use of for the purpose, and sometimes a pair of hand bellows have been used; but I would prefer the breath, as most likely to keep the lungs and blood warm.

P. Smith, 1812

LIVER

TO RELIEVE DISTRESS

The juice of ½ lemon in a glass of hot water, without sugar, taken night and morning will do wonders for an inactive liver. It excites the torpid organ, stimulates the digestive apparatus, and tones up the general system.

To 1 pint hot water add the juice of 1 lemon and ½ teaspoon salt. Sip this ½ hour before breakfast every morning for 2 weeks, then skip 2 weeks. This is especially beneficial if taken during the months of March and April.

A decoction of either the leaves or bark of maple tree is good to strengthen the liver. It is also good to ease pains in the sides, which proceed from the liver and spleen.

Make a strong tea of snake's head herb, and drink freely.

Liverwort is a good herb for the liver. It is to be given in strong decoction.

Steep heaping teaspoon of Rocky Mountain grape root in 1 cup of boiling water. Strain when cold. Take a wineglassful after each meal.

Mrs. G., 1952

A decoction of black alder bark removes obstructions in the liver and spleen, and removes the hardness of the former.

Wild celandine cleanses the liver and spleen, and opens the urinary passage.

St. John's wort herb has a particular influence on the liver; its tea is an excellent remedy for it. A small admixture of aloe powder increases the effect, which can be observed chiefly in the urine.

Old German recipe

Joepye roots steeped in boiling water, and drunk cold corrects the bile.

More than a 100 cases have been cured either by the simple extract of dandelion herb and root, or by taking a teacupful of a strong decoction twice a day.

Dandelion root is one of the finest medicines known for bilious complaints, and can easily be made into pills. Those who have long been habituated to swallowing a pill or 2 every night will find this as healthy a kind as they can use.

P. F. Bowker, 1836

Take 2 pounds of dandelion roots and tops, when green, pound them and add 1 pint of liquor, strain it, and take ⅔ of a wineglass 1 morning, and a glass of spring water the next, so continue for 9 mornings, and it will relieve the complaint. (Try it.) Or take 1 pound of dandelions, pound them so as to get the juice, take 2 pounds water cresses, simmer them together, add ½ ounce licorice and ½ pint of gin; take ½ wineglassful 3 times a day.

Dr. L. Sperry, 1843

Make a strong tea or syrup of dandelion, burdock root and wormwood herb, and drink freely in small doses.

Take equal parts of wild yam, black root, sacred bark, fringe tree, boldo leaves, and dandelion root. Mix ingredients. Steep heaping teaspoon in 1 cup of boiling water until cool. Take wineglass-ful morning and night.

M. G., Nurse, 1961

Take equal parts of yarrow herb, agrimony herb, goldenrod, wild carrot herb, germander herb, pellitory-of-the-wall, broom herb and dandelion. Mix ingredients thoroughly. Use 1 teaspoon of mixture to each cup of boiling water. Strain when cold. Dose 2 table-spoons after each meal.

Syrup for a person that is troubled with a bilious habit. Take dande-lion root and branch [slice up], and bark from the root of a poplar, equal parts; boil these in water till the strength is all out, then strain it off and simmer it down till it becomes quite thick; add while warm 1 gill of molasses to a pint of syrup. If in warm weather, add a very little gin to keep it from souring. Take a teaspoon 3 times a day for a dose. This for a person troubled with a bilious habit is one of the best things known, for it is perfectly harmless and does not weaken in the operation.

Bitters to go with the above syrup. Take bitter root, poplar bark, and the leaves of snake's head and barberry bark, equal parts; dry these and pound them fine; sift them through a fine sieve; take a teaspoon of this in a wineglassful of warm water, sweetened, every morning before eating.

P. F. Bowker, 1836

CHRONIC LIVER COMPLAINT

Take of golden seal, bitter root, blue flag root, mayapple root, each in coarse powder, a tablespoon; bloodroot ½ tablespoon; red pepper, a teaspoon; whisky 2 pints; mix; let them stand 10 or 12 days, frequently shaking, and sweeten if desired. The dose is 1 or 2 tea-spoons 3 or 4 times a day, or enough to produce 1 operation from the bowels every day.

Take of Indian turnip, elecampane root, and comfrey roots, each, in coarse powder, ½ tablespoon; horseradish root, yellow parilla root, hoarhound leaves, and black cohosh, each, in coarse powder 1 tablespoon; whisky or spirits 1 quart; mix; let them stand 10 or 12 days, frequently shaking, and sweeten if desired. The dose is a tablespoon 3 or 4 times a day.

Take of the green herb *Lycopus europaeus* 2 parts; fresh inner bark of hickory, and fresh inner bark of white ash, coarsely bruised, 1 part; fill a gallon jug with these, and fill with whisky; let it stand 5 or 6 days, frequently shaking. The dose is a tablespoon 3 or 4 times a day. This is especially useful in liver and spleen affections which follow chills and fever.

J. King, M.D., 1864

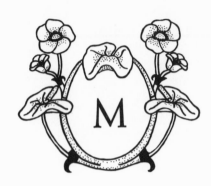

MEASLES

Measles generally requires but little medical treatment. The patient should be placed in a large well-ventilated room, and it is better that he should remain in bed. He *should not* be given warm drinks, or emetics, as they only tend to increase the fever. Of cold water he may have all he desires. The diet should be light, such as wheat or rice flour gruel, toast water, milk and water, tapioca, sago, or other light food. He may be allowed a more liberal diet as the fever decreases. The eyes should be shaded from the light.

Diet for this complaint ought to be low: such as mush and boiled milk, chicken soup, etc. The drinks are to be slippery elm tea, flaxseed tea, balm tea, etc. Nothing to be taken cold or hot, but moderately warm.

Give child all the lemonade (warm or cool) it can drink and keep in a warm room. Do not give cold drinks too frequently.

An infusion made of elder berry blossoms is good to drive out the measles. Tea may be sweetened.

Hot chamomile is used to bring out the rash of measles.

Marigold flowers may be taken in simple infusion. Place 1 ounce in a vessel and pour 1 pint of boiling water. Allow to cool. This can be freely drunk by all ages. Sweeten with honey if necessary.

Take a quantity of common nettles, steep them strong, let the patient drink freely of the juice, and it will drive them out, when nothing else will. This is the Irish way of curing this disease.

Pleurisy root is a specific in measles, being far superior to saffron.

Take a wineglassful of vervain tea 3 times a day, as a preventative. When the disease shows itself, place the feet of the patient in warm water and mustard, and give plentifully of vervain; keep a fire in the room to prevent chills, and be sure to attend to the bowels; if costive, give a dose of senna and ginger tea.

MENSES

SUPPRESSED, OBSTRUCTED, SCANTY

A hot foot bath is often all that is necessary.

Keep bowels open; ride horseback, or moderate exercise. Good Madeira wine, taken frequently in small quantities; bitters, made of equal quantities of wild cherry bark and poplar bark, steeped in wine several days, and taken in moderate doses; or tea made of the flowers of chamomile, and taken cold, in doses of a wineglassful, 3 or 4 times a day. The chalybeate water should be used freely. The western country abounds with these waters; for they are to be found on almost every branch or creek. Chalybeate waters are those springs which are impregnated with iron.

J. C. Gunn, M.D., 1830

Drink a hot tea made of Jamaica ginger before retiring or drink a wineglassful of tea made of wild ginger root 2 or 3 times a day.

Drink a hot tea 3 times a day, made with 1 teaspoon of marjoram herb steeped in 1 cup of boiling water.

Drink a hot tea made of fennel seeds 3 times a day.

Drink infusion made of wintergreen leaves several times a day.

Boil 1 ounce of the herb female regulator in 1 pint of water for a couple of minutes and strain. Dose, take small doses of a tablespoonful 4 or 5 times a day.

An infusion of top and flowers of tansy taken in small doses is excellent in producing menstruation when for any reason the flow is retarded.

Smartweed herb has been used extensively by women of this country for promoting the menses.

An infusion made with juniper berries promotes the monthly terms of woman.

Take a strong tea made of seneca snakeroot, as much as the stomach will bear. Another source advises administering to the extent of 4 ounces of the decoction in the course of the day, increased as the menstrual effort is expected.

In cases of sudden suppression of the menses, a tumbler full of pennyroyal tea with a level teaspoon of black pepper pounded fine, sweetened, and drunk warm after soaking the feet in weak lye, will rarely fail of producing the desired effect.

The hot tea of boneset herb is an efficacious medicine in suppressions of the menstrual function. Besides the profuse sweat which it excites, it relaxes the vessels of the uterus, and operates upon that organ as it does upon the skin.

G. Capron, M.D., and C. B. Slack, M.D., 1848

Steep a handful of blood roots in ½ pint of old whiskey, letting it stand 5 or 8 days, when the tincture is fit for use—beginning with 10 drops, and gradually increasing the dose, as circumstances may require. To give in decoction or tea use a handful of roots to a quart of boiling water—a tablespoon every 2 or 3 hours, as required.

Take of smartweed, wild sage or cancerweed, vervain and pennyroyal each equal parts. Fill a jug or bottle with them, and then add as much whisky as the vessel will hold. Let it stand a few days, frequently shaking, when it will be fit for use. Dose, a tablespoon 3 or 4 times a day, in ½ gill sweetened water.

Take of horseradish root, calamus root, motherwort herb, blue cohosh root, each, coarsely bruised, an ounce; whisky 3 pints; mix, let it stand 10 or 12 days, frequently shaking. Dose, same as the preceding.

Motherwort herb is one of the most useful herbs to relieve obstructed menstruation.

Mrs. A. Matteson, 1894

In order to help the discharge, take 1 teaspoon of the tincture of gum guaiacum in a tumbler of new milk on going to bed, 2 or 3 nights before the full of the moon; and at the same time make a strong tea of snakeroot and drink in the course of the day as much as the stomach will bear. This may be depended upon as an infallible remedy.

Dr. A. A. Benezet, 1826

Make a tea from 2 teaspoons quassia to 1 pint of water. Drink when cold the night before the flow should start. It will never fail if taken up to a month after it works.

Mrs. T. Robinson, 1931

The best and most powerful medicines for the regulation of retained or obstructed menses may be found upon almost any farm in New England. The first article which we shall name is the savin. The tops and leaves of this tree, ground into a powder, or made into a tea, and taken or drunk in a sufficient quantity to raise a perspiration, for several days in succession, have been ascertained to produce the menstrual effusion in 4 cases out of 5. The dose in powder, which is the best way of giving it, is a scruple at a time. It should be given at least 3 times a day. The next medicine whose virtues are established in the regulation of the menstrual effusion, is the red century. A strong tea should be made of it, and copious draughts of it taken hot, every hour or every 2 hours, at such times as nature appears to be making an effort, until a moisture is produced upon the skin.

G. Capron, M.D., and D. B. Slack, M.D., 1848

PAINFUL, DIFFICULT MENSES; CRAMPS

When the attack commences, take a warm hip-bath: lie in bed and apply cloths wrung out of water to the lower part of the abdomen. Drink a decoction of blue cohosh several times a day, ½ or ⅓ cupful at a time.

Painful menses is often brought on by colds. Treat by warm hip-baths, hot drinks (avoiding spirituous liquors), and heat applied to the back and extremities. A teaspoon of the fluid extract of viburnum will sometimes act like a charm.

Drink freely of tea made of red raspberry leaves.

Take 4 parts red raspberry leaves, 1 part skunk cabbage root, 1 part ginger. Steep tablespoon of the mixture in 1 cup of boiling water. Strain and drink when moderately warm as often as needed.

The hot infusion of chamomile flowers, in full dosage is quite effective in dysmenorrhea, especially the non-obstructive type. Indeed, this agent is often more effective than valerian—certainly it is more agreeable in the uterine reflex disturbances of women.

Take 5 or 10 drops of oil of chamomile on a loaf of sugar.

The decoction made from the bark of the root of cotton plant was used by slaves for painful and obstructed menses.

Drink freely of an infusion made with hops.

A tea of thyme, drunk warm, is useful.

Put a small teacup of logwood chips in a pint of soft water, simmer 15 minutes, then add ½ pint of whisky. Dose, 1 tablespoon ½ hour before each meal and just before going to bed.

Practical Housekeeping, 1887

Take 2 teaspoons of dried wormwood and 2 teaspoons of pennyroyal, steep in a cup of boiling water for 2 or 3 minutes. Strain and drink while hot.

Mrs. C. Tharp

Take of pennyroyal a handful; steep in a pint of boiling water for ½ hour; then add 4 teaspoons of powdered cinnamon, and a heaping teaspoon of powdered borax; when the borax is dissolved, it may be sweetened. Dose, ½ gill every hour or 2 until the menses come on and the pain is relieved.

J. King, M.D., 1864

PROFUSE, EXCESSIVE

Avoid highly seasoned food and the use of spirituous liquors; also excessive fatigue, either physical or mental. To check the flow, patient should be kept quiet, and allowed to sip cinnamon tea during the period.

Maintain a recumbent position, use plain diet, and abstain from all stimulating food and drinks. The feet must be soaked in warm water, and cold cloths applied to the lower parts of the abdomen. Give 1 or 2 teaspoons every 2 or 3 hours in sweetened water the following mixture: oil of cinnamon 2 drachms, oil of erigeron 1 drachm, pulverized gum arabic 1 drachm, water 4 ounces.

S. Pancoast, M.D., 1901

Take yarrow and shepherd's purse, each, a handful of the fresh plants; boiling water 1½ pints; mix. Steep in a covered vessel near fire, for ½ hour; when cold, give ½ gill 3 or 4 times a day. This will be found a superior remedy.

Equal parts of black haw and wild alum root made into decoction. Drink as needed.

A. Burch

Mix the following in powdered form; 1 ounce cranesbill root; 2 ounces white poplar bark; 1 ounce bistort root; 1 ounce golden seal root; ½ ounce cloves; ¼ ounce ginger; ½ pound ground sugar. Dose, 1 teaspoon in a ½ cup of boiling water 3 times a day.

Amaranth or prince's feather is most celebrated as a remedy for profuse menstruation, and has often cured when other remedies have failed.

H. Howard, 1857

Take 1 ounce powdered witch hazel; 1 ounce powdered bayberry; ¼ ounce powdered ginger. Mix thoroughly. Place 1 or 2 teaspoons in a glass of hot milk and sip 2 or 3 times during the day.

Douche for excessive flowing: make a strong decoction of equal parts of raspberry leaves and witch hazel.

REGULATORS (FOLK TERM)

Squaw weed seems to have a special and very favorable influence upon the female organs of generation—so much so that it has acquired the name of female regulator. In its sensible action it is diuretic, tonic, diaphoretic and pectoral; but is mainly used and most useful for its action upon the uterus. In all cases of obstructed or suppressed menses, it is highly valuable, either alone, or in combination with wild ginger or vervain root, to be taken in tea or infusion. In cases of painful or too profuse menstruation, and in flooding from the womb, or menorrhagia, combined with the cinnamon bark and raspberry leaves, it is also extremely valuable taken freely in infusion.

J. C. Gunn, M.D., 1862

For suppressed, painful or excessive menstruation, take from 10 to 30 grains of the powdered star root 3 times a day, in ordinary cases; in urgent cases, as in dysmenorrhea, flooding, and the like, it should be given in doses of ½ teaspoon, in a little hot water, once an hour or oftener, until several doses are taken. The dose of the infusion is about ½ a teacupful, repeated according to circumstances.

Jill-grow-over-the-ground is the best thing known in the world to correct female irregularities.

P. F. Bowker, 1836

Mugwort is a friend to break up the vicious circle of perverted menstrual function in cases of dysmenorrhea, the stops and starts of amenorrhea. It affords remarkable symptomatic relief by raising the tone of the musculature of the uterus and by sustaining utero-circulation. Over a few months its use promotes a healthy menstrual cycle.

CHANGE OF LIFE (MENOPAUSE)

There is no better herb than mother-wort for cleansing the womb and removing obstructions in the female at this time of life. A wineglassful of the decoction should be taken 3 times a day.

Excessive flowing in change of life: Grate 1 ounce of nutmeg in 1 pint Jamaica rum, mix well. Dose, 1 teaspoon 3 times a day as long as necessary.

Equal parts of white plantain, sumac leaves, yellow dock, or burdock and devil's bit. Boil them and sweeten with molasses and put ¼ part spirits. Dose, a wineglass ½ full 3 times a day. Good for all female derangements, specially at the change. Called mother's friend

Dr. B. W. James, 1852

MOUTH

Also see THROAT.

BAD BREATH

In children it generally indicates a disordered stomach or loaded bowels when not caused by decayed teeth or morbid secretion of the tonsils. A tumbler of chamomile tea on rising every morning often corrects this condition.

Infuse a handful of raspberry leaves in a ½ pint of boiling water for 15 minutes; when cold strain, and add 2 ounces of the tincture of myrrh. Rinse the mouth with a little of it 2 or 3 times a day, swallowing a little each time, until relieved.

Chew 1 or 2 whole cloves, cardamon seeds, or a whole cubeb.

CANKER OR THRUSH

Take a piece of alum, rub on the canker often.

Burn a corn cob and apply the ashes on the sores 2 or 3 times a day.

Take 4 large spoonfuls of good cider vinegar, 4 of water, 1 teaspoon of salt and a very small portion of black or red pepper. Gargle or swab the mouth. (Pepper may be left out.)

The most important thing is to keep the mouth of the child clean. A few grains of borax dissolved in a teacup of water and used as a wash after each feeding will generally be effective. A very nice application is to dissolve ½ drachm of borax with 1 drachm of glycerin and 1 ounce of water.

Rinse the mouth well with a weak solution of borax on canker.

Take ½ teaspoon borax, ½ teaspoon tincture of myrrh, 1 teaspoon glycerine and enough boiled water to make 1 ounce. Apply gently to the inside of the mouth several times a day with clean camel's hair brush.

Swab the mouth out with a little borax and honey, and occasionally a little raspberry leaf tea, keeping the bowels moderately open with the soothing syrup.

Infuse a handful of raspberry leaves in ½ pint of boiling water for 15 minutes; when cold strain and add 2 ounces tincture of myrrh, rinse the mouth with a little of it 2 or 3 times a day, swallow a little each time until relieved.

Black currant jelly is an excellent remedy for canker and sore mouth. Pick your currants clean, mash them, stew them and rub through a sieve; add the same weight of loaf sugar, and simmer over a slow fire 30 or 35 minutes.

A tea made of the ripe berries of sumach and sweetened with honey is good for canker in the mouth. It is also used as a gargle, in putrid fevers, to remove the thrush and sores from the mouth and teeth.

G. Capron, M.D., and D. B. Slack, M.D., 1848

Make a strong decoction of 1 tablespoon each of sumach bark and white oak bark, add a piece of alum as big as a hazelnut. Boil in a quart of water. Use as mouth wash or gargle.

Equal quantity of sweet apple tree bark, blackberry root, bark of root of sumach, and borax. Steep in water.

Grandma Allen's Recipe Book, about 1820

Take sage, hyssop, sumac berries, equal parts: make a strong decoction, sweeten with honey, and to ½ a pint of it add ½ teaspoon pulverized borax: let the mouth be often washed with this.

Take the yolk of a roasted egg, burnt leather, sage pulverized, and burnt alum, mix with honey. It will cure canker or sore mouth.

Cleanse the mouth with a little sage tea sweetened with honey and mixed with a dram of borax. If the canker sore affects the throat great benefit may be derived from a decoction of carrots in water. Sweeten with honey and give several times a day.

Take the scrapings of a blackberry briar root, a little saffron, a little sage, and some gold thread, or yellow root. Put with these a little alum, some vinegar and honey, simmer this on hot ashes, after adding a little water. Wet the mouth often. It seldom fails of a cure.

Take plantain leaves, honeysuckles, sage and rosemary, equal parts, and boil them in sour wine, add thereto a little honey and alum. Wash the mouth with this as often as necessary. A few times will be sufficient. It is very harmless, but not more so than it is healing.

Take of plantain seeds 1 ounce, boil in 1½ pints of water, down to 1 pint. Strain and sweeten with honey. Give 1 tablespoon 3 or 4 times a day.

Make a tea from common strawberry leaves. This may be used to swab baby's mouth. Add a small piece of alum to the infusion for adults.

Make a strong decoction of red oak bark, add a little salt and pepper. Use as a gargle. Do not add pepper if parts are very red and inflamed.

Chew a small twig from a cherry tree, letting the bruised bark rest on the sore spot. Relief is generally immediate and mouth heals quickly.

Mrs. C. Bigelow, Nurse, 1917

To relieve thrush in infants who are still nursing, the mother may chew small pieces of rhubarb root. Two or 3 pieces the size of a pea every day. This often benefits the infant through the mother's milk.

Goldthread roots, made into a strong tea, thickened with cream, and made sweet with loaf sugar, and applied with a swab, made of a linen rag, tied on the end of a stick, is good.

A decoction of quince seed makes a soothing gargle in aphthous affections, and ulcerations of the mouth. The decoction is made in following manner: take 2 drachms quince seed to 1 pint of water. Boil them over gentle heat for 10 minutes and strain.

English recipe

A strong decoction of marsh rosemary is good for canker.

A decoction of golden seal root and blue cohosh, used as a wash or gargle is useful in ulcerated sore mouth and throat. Another: make a decoction of yarrow herb or privet bush leaves and beth root; sweeten with honey.

Wash the mouth frequently with some warm astringent infusion as the following: Equal parts goldenseal, cranesbill root, alum; or infusion made with red root, witch hazel bark, and cranesbill.

Drink an infusion made with hops. Hold it in the mouth several minutes before swallowing.

MISCELLANEOUS MOUTH COMPLAINTS

When chewed, ginger root excites the salivary glands, and hence it has been found useful in relaxations of the uvula and tonsils; and paralysis of the tongue and fauces.

Scurvy in the mouth: Take prince-of-pine or scurvy grass, boil it in water, add to it rum and honey, hold it in the mouth as hot as it can be borne, and boil a large quantity of herbs, and sweat the head over it.

GUMS

Gumboils: Wash them out with warm water, adding ½ teaspoon tincture of myrrh and a pinch of saleratus to each cup of water.

Spongy gums: Rub with tincture of myrrh.

Denture-sore gums: Rub with tincture of myrrh or with gel of aloe vera.

LIPS

Take 4 parts lard, 2 parts white wax, 2 parts spermaceti; melt, and work well together. Pour into little glass boxes. Perfume if you like.

Take 2 tablespoons of sweet oil, a piece of beeswax the size of a hazelnut, melt over a lamp, in a piece of letter paper large enough to hold it.

Sore lips: Wash lips with a strong decoction made from the bark of white oak.

MUMPS

In this disorder the patient should not expose himself to take cold in the damp air, or by wetting his feet, but should continually have recourse to stimulating spirits, and bathe the swelling with the same. If the patient should swell downwards, take white beans, pound them fine, and make a poultice of them in milk and water, and apply to the swelling. If this should not check the swelling, take the garden chamomile and simmer it in milk, and with the liquor bathe the part affected, and drink infusions of the herb. A wash made of the roots and tops of bittersweet is likewise an excellent remedy, and should be taken internally, and applied externally.

J. Monroe, 1824

A mild infusion of scullcap tea will work wonders. Two teaspoons scullcap herb should be placed in a teacup and boiling water poured on. Add 3 or 4 drops oil of spearmint if recovery is a little tardy. For children under 7, give 2 to 3 teaspoons 4 times daily, and for those above this age, ½ to 1 teacupful. Hot fomentations of chamomile flowers applied over the swollen area will assist in reducing the swelling.

In ordinary cases, the disease is mild, and requires only a little good nursing, and care that the body be kept warm and dry. The child should stay in the house, and if the swellings are painful use hot herb teas, such as pennyroyal, peppermint, or catnip in order to cause sweat. A large, thick piece of flannel, or, which is better, a clean woolen sock, should be worn around the neck, and the food should consist of rye pudding or brown bread, with sweetened water. If the swellings and inflammation become severe, cathartics, and sudorifics will be required.

G. Capron, M.D., and D. B. Slack, M.D., 1848

For pain, bathe parts with mixture of 1 dram scraped castile soap, ½ ounce oil of sassafras, 1 ounce olive oil, 3 drams camphor. Warm this mixture and apply 3 times a day.

Apply to the swelling 1 part each of lobelia extract, oil of mustard and tincture of myrrh and 3 parts camphor. After applying, cover with warm flannel.

MUSCULAR CRAMPS

When cramps attack the muscles of the legs, relief may often be obtained by exciting the opposite muscles in action.

Tie a piece of cotton cloth tight above the pain, then wear a piece of cotton cloth well rubbed with flower of sulphur around the ankle.

Wrap legs in towels wrung out in cold water, and put on the outside a thick dry cloth.

As soon as you feel the cramp coming, raise the toes upward and the cramp will leave immediately.

Try setting the feet squarely on something cold.

Steep 1 teaspoon cranberry bush bark in 1 cup of boiling water for 5 or 10 minutes. Drink 2 or 3 times a day for cramps in legs or other parts of the body.

Letter, 1958

Rub oil of wintergreen on painful parts.

Take 1 part oil of peppermint and 2 parts alcohol and apply on affected parts.

Rub painful parts with oil of turpentine.

Rub parts with mixture of camphorated oil, turpentine and spirits of hartshorn.

Take 1 gallon alcohol, 1 ounce oil cajaput, 1 ounce oil of monarda, 1 ounce oil of thyme, ½ ounce oil of peppermint, 1 ounce camphor gum. Shake well and let stand 24 hours. Good for man or beast.

Rub a little opodeldoc upon the part affected, 2 or 3 times a day, and wear a flannel upon it; if this does not give relief, take 20 drops of volatile tincture of guaiacum every night and morning, in a glass of spring water.

Recipe for opodeldoc: Take of Hungary-water a pint; Castile soap sliced, 3 ounces; camphor, an ounce; let them stand together in a glass closely stopped, till the soap and camphor are entirely dissolved in the Hungary-water.

H. L. Barnum, 1831

NAUSEA

SEA OR CAR SICKNESS

The white of an egg and the juice of 1 lemon, well beaten together and slightly sweetened, if taken just before starting for a car ride, will prevent car sickness.

Travelers who are much troubled with indigestion and nausea, should never forget to take with them as a faithful companion their little bottle of wormwood tincture.

Take as much cayenne pepper as you can bear in a bowl of hot soup and, it is said, all sickness, nausea and squeamishness will disappear.

For sea sickness, drink copiously of strong green tea as often as the stomach will bear it. It is simple, but effective.

Drink a weak infusion of chamomile tea.

A teaspoon of essence of peppermint in a glass of hot water, sip occasionally.

Chew a leaf or 2 of mint or sage to a tasteless pulp.

NERVOUSNESS

Nervous people are greatly benefited by a diet of celery. Onions are next best. Parsley and vinegar removes the effects of eating onions. No medicine is really so efficacious in case of nervous prostration, and they tone up a wornout system in a very short time.

Miss M. C. Cooke, 1889

Motherwort herb is without doubt, as useful an herb as grows for women. It is good for all nervous and hypochondriac affections, dizziness in the head, and a strong tea made of this and drunk freely, will raise the drooping spirits, and give new vigor to the whole system.

Lady slipper root is used by the Indians in all nervous disorders. It is called perfectly harmless. It may be given in hysterical symptoms, spasmodic affections, and all disorders of the nerves. It answers a much better purpose than opium, for it has a tendency to quiet the nerves without destroying sensibility. It may be given in boiling water, sweetened, something like ½ teaspoon at a dose. You will find this to answer the most sanguine expectations.

The following varieties of lady slipper are most efficient for nervous disorders: *Cypripedium luteum; C. acaule; C. spectabile; C. candidum.*

C. S. Rafinesque, 1828

Boil a tablespoon of hops in a pint of water for a few minutes. Allow it to steep 5 minutes and strain. Drink small doses frequently.

A tea made of catnip herb is very quieting, especially for nervous women. May also be given to children.

Chew root of ginseng and swallow the juice.

Take equal parts of mistletoe, scullcap herb, valerian root, and wood betony herb, mix. Use 1 ounce of the mixture to 1 pint of water. Boil for 5 minutes. Strain when cool. Drink wineglassful 3 times a day.

NEURALGIA

Lemon eaten freely, without the peel and without sugar, has proved very beneficial.

Half a drachm of sal ammoniac in 1 ounce of camphor water, to be taken a teaspoon at a dose, and the dose repeated several times, at intervals of 5 minutes, if the pain be not relieved at once.

A decoction made of the roots of bull nettle will give relief from neuralgia. Drink a wineglassful 2 or 3 times a day.

Take 1 cupful of smartweed, simmer for 10 minutes in a quart of water. Take ½ cup of the hot decoction, sweetened with honey, every hour, or more if pain is severe.

Steep 1 ounce of burdock seeds in a pint of boiling water 1 hour. Strain and take 1 tablespoon before meals and at bed time.

Mrs. M. Finley, 1916

Pour 1 pint of boiling water over 1 ounce of scullcap herb. Cover and allow to steep until cold. Strain and take a wineglassful every hour or 2.

Drink freely of tea made of parsley leaves.

Gather Canada thistles when in flower and dry. Turn boiling water on a quantity of the thistles, let steep 5 or 10 minutes, turn out and sweeten to taste. Before drinking it fix for a sweat in a warm room, then drink of the tea while it is hot in large quantities. Follow taking the tea for a few days, and you will effect a cure; do not drink it hot after the sweat, but either warm or cold.

Miss T. S. Shute, 1878

EXTERNAL APPLICATIONS

A towel folded several times and dipped in hot water and quickly wrung and applied over the seat of the pain generally affords prompt relief.

A small bag of hot salt applied to the pain, or apply cloth steeped in hot vinegar.

Cut a lemon or 2 and squeeze juice on parts afflicted and rub in, then place hot cloths over it.

Neuralgia of head and face may often be relieved by the application of a spice plaster of ginger, cinnamon, cloves, etc., instead of the usual mustard plaster.

Horseradish leaves wilted and bound on cures neuralgia.

Grate horseradish root and mix it in vinegar, the same as for table purposes, and apply to the temple when the face or the head is affected, or the wrist when the pain is in the arm or shoulder.

Mash the leaves of plantain and apply to sore spot.

Mrs. R. C., 1952

Boil a small handful of lobelia in ½ pint of water till the strength is out of the herb, then strain it off and add a teaspoon of fine salt. Wring cloths out of the liquid as hot as possible, and spread over the part affected. It acts like a charm. Change the cloths as soon as cold till the pain is all gone; then cover the place with a soft dry covering till perspiration is over, to prevent taking cold. Rheumatism can often be relieved by application to the painful parts, of cloths wet in a weak solution of sal soda water. If there is inflammation in the joints the cure is very quick. The wash should be lukewarm.

Macerate the leaves of the common field thistle and use a poultice on the parts affected, while a small quantity of the same is boiled down to the proportion of 1 quart to 1 pint, and a small wine-glassful of the decoction drunk before each meal. A friend says he has never known it to fail of giving relief, while in almost every case it has effected a cure.

Mrs. M. W. Ellsworth, 1897

NIGHT SWEATS

Put 1 or more basins of water under the bed of the patient, and renew every day. A change for the better will be observed in a very short time. Another suggestion is to have a strong, healthy person occupy the bed with the patient for a few nights.

Mrs. Owens' New Cook Book, 1897

Drink freely of an infusion made of sage.

Bathe the body in salt water every other day. Just before retiring take a cup of sage tea, and eat nourishing foods.

NOSE

NOSEBLEED

Raise the arm on the same side as that of the nostril from which the blood flows.

Hold both arms above the head.

Put the feet into water as hot as can be borne, keep them there until relieved. This draws the blood from the head.

Soak the feet and hands in warm soapsuds, or water. Apply a cloth wrung out in cold water on the back of the neck, and on the cords behind the ears.

Stand perfectly erect, throw the head a little back, place the finger on the affected side of the nose, close the mouth tightly and draw air through the free nostril as long as possible. Repeat this until the bleeding ceases. Vigorous chewing motion of the jaws will arrest bleeding at the nose. If necessary take a wad of paper and chew hard.

Place the finger on the side of the nose, tightly, for 10 or 15 minutes.

Put pieces of ice in cloths and lay one on each side of the nose and 1 on the back of the neck.

Apply cold water to face and back of neck and sniff powdered alum.

Wet a cloth in cold water and strong vinegar and apply to back of neck.

Place a piece of writing paper on the gums of the upper jaw, under the upper lip, and let it remain there for a few minutes.

A wedge of salt pork inserted in the nose.

Take a piece of very dry and hard salt beef, that which has been smoked is best, and grate it into a powder, and push of this up the nostrils, as far as possible, until they are filled, and let it remain until it stops. This never fails.

Bathe the feet in very hot water, drinking at the same time a pint of cayenne pepper tea.

Gum arabic, powdered fine and sniffed from your fingers, or blown into the nose through a quill is good.

Get some fresh mullein leaves, pound them and sniff the juice up the nostrils. It has proven very effective.

A snuff made of the leaves of witch hazel, and inhaled into the nose will, in most cases, stop the bleeding. Wetting the face, and temples, at the same time with cold water, will assist the effects of the hazel. A tea of hazel, with the addition of cayenne, will also be beneficial, taken internally; to which may likewise be added the common beth root, either in tea or substance, or it may be taken alone, in a larger quantity.

Take nosebleed and horsetail, dry them, and pulverize fine. Sniff this for nosebleed.

Make a strong infusion of horsetail and sniff up the nostrils.

A constant drink of the infusion of yarrow herb for 3 days, prevents the nosebleed for a year.

Take common nettle roots, dry them, and chew them every day as you would tobacco. Continue this 3 weeks.

OBSTRUCTIONS IN THE NOSE

Cause sneezing by sniffing snuff or by tickling the nose with a feather. If these fail, a hair-pin or shoe-button-hook may be carefully tried.

The Housewife's Library, 1885

When a child has any substance wedged in its nostrils, press the vacant nostril so as to close it, and apply your lips close to the child's mouth and blow very hard. This simple method will generally force the substance out of the nostril.

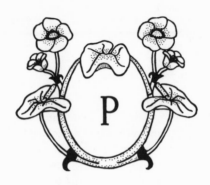

PAIN

To relieve pain from wounds, take a pan or shovel with burning coals and sprinkle upon them common brown sugar, and hold the wounded part in the smoke. In a few minutes the pain will be allayed, and recovery proceeds rapidly.

Make a brine as strong as you can, add 1 ounce of capsicum in boiling water, till it draws sufficiently and then mix them and put 1 pint of alcohol. Ready for use.

The leaves of horsebalm are famous for raising sweat wherever a bunch of them is applied to the skin, and by that means give ease of pain in any part where they are applied. Apply a bunch of them to a stiff neck, bind them close, it will raise a sweat and effect a cure.

For pain in the spine, mix beef gall with vinegar, and bathe the back with the wash night and morning.

Steep marigold flowers in good cider vinegar, and frequently wash the affected parts; this will afford speedy relief; or take ½ of white pine tar and ½ pound tobacco, and boil them down separately to a thick substance, then simmer them together; spread a plaster and apply it to the affected parts, and it will afford immediate relief.

Take of alcohol, 1 quart, and add equal quantities of the oils of wormwood, tansy, white or red cedar, and hemlock, as much as the spirits will dissolve; then add 1 pint of sharp vinegar, and a tablespoon of cayenne. This is to be applied externally in cases of pains and swellings.

EXTERNAL AND INTERNAL

Put 1 tablespoon cayenne pepper in a wide-mouthed bottle, add ½ pint pure alcohol and a small piece of camphor. Cork and let stand 12 or 14 days. This is an excellent internal and external remedy. One teaspoon is a dose for internal use.

To 1 gallon of alcohol add ¼ pound of gum myrrh, ¼ pound of gum guaiacum, ½ ounce oil of wintergreen, ½ ounce red pepper. Mix and let it stand until the gums are dissolved. Good for all pains. Dose, 10 drops in water, and rub well on parts affected.

S. Thomson, 1831

For pains in muscles or bones, drink freely of decoction made with roots of wisteria [*Wisteria sinensis*].

PHLEGM

Take the leaves of colt's foot, dry them, and use them as you would tobacco for smoking. This simple remedy has not been known to fail of giving relief in any instance where it has been used.

Fresh nettles just gathered, dried and made into tea, loosen the phlegm in the chest and lungs, cleanse the stomach from matters gathered there, which they expel chiefly by means of the kidneys.

Mallow flowers prepared as tea, loosens the phlegm on the chest. The blossoms may be mixed with mullein flowers.

The dried leaves of ribwort yield likewise a splendid tea against interior phlegm obstructions.

A tea made with sage removes phlegm from the palate, throat, or stomach.

Prepared as a tea, rosemary cleanses the stomach from phlegm, gives a good appetite and good digestion.

Tea made from the leaves of chicory removes phlegm from the stomach.

Blue violet leaves taken as tea assist in loosening the phlegm of consumptive people.

PILES or HEMORRHOIDS

Make a wash of vinegar and water and apply frequently.

When piles are much inflamed use a poultice made of the common smoking tobacco and fresh butter, in the proportion of 1 part of the former to 2 of the latter, simmered and strained, to be applied 2 or 3 times a day.

If piles are external, rub on linseed oil; or, if internal, take a teaspoon of the same, 3 times a day; or, take of sulphur 1 ounce, hog's fat 4 ounces, strong tobacco juice ½ pint, and simmer them together into an ointment; and apply it.

Take a heaping teaspoon of milk of sulphur before retiring; also wash the parts with strong borax water, injecting if possible, and apply a soft linen cloth well saturated with the solution. Repeat once or twice until a cure is effected.

Mix a teaspoon of flour of sulphur with a teacup of milk, and take twice a day, morning and night, until improvement takes place, then take occasionally.

Apply 3 times daily dry flour of sulphur to the parts. If it will not adhere mix with sweet oil or vaseline as a salve.

Steep a teaspoon of whole flaxseed in a pint of boiling water for about 5 minutes or longer, then strain. When lukewarm inject it into rectum as an enema.

Oil anus night and morning with almond oil. Place a peeled clove of garlic in the rectum overnight. Rest every day for ½ hour, with pillow under the small of the back, but none at the head, 3 times a day. Take a natural squatting position at stool.

The bark of white pine should be boiled and the soft part stript out and beat to a poultice in a mortar, and then sufficiently moistened with the liquor in which it was boiled. Apply with a feather. Drink a little tea made of the bark.

Take equal parts of the pitch of white pine and fir balsam, make this into pills, and take 4 or 5 per day.

Take 1 gill of molasses, 1 ounce of fresh butter, mix them well over a slow fire, and drink, just before lying down, or going to bed at night. In addition to this, the following external application should be made. Burn 2 common sized new corks to ashes, and mix the same with a sufficient quantity of lard to make it of proper consistence; rub the anus or fundament twice a day with this ointment, and a cure will soon be effected.

For internal use, boil 1 ounce of yellow dock root in 1½ pints of water. Strain. Dose, a wineglassful night and morning. Make an ointment of 4 ounces pure lard [not salted], 1 ounce of the leaves of plantain, ½ ounce leaves of ground ivy. Place all together in an enamelled pan and simmer over gentle heat for about 10 minutes. Press leaves well in the lard to get out all the goodness; strain into a jar and use when cool. Put the ointment freely into the rectum at night. The decoction of yellow dock and ointment may be used at the same time.

Gipsy recipe

Take 4 ripe buckeyes or horse chestnuts, while still fresh, carefully remove the outer brownish shell from them, and slice them up finely. Put them into a tin cup with a sufficient quantity of melted lard to cover them, and let them steep near a fire for an hour. Then strain and press out the lard, and when cool it is fit for use. A portion of this ointment must be applied to the pile tumors and within the lower bowel twice every day.

J. King, M.D., 1864

Take the whole plant of wild lettuce, cut up and boil in suitable quantity of water for an hour, then strain and press out all the juice, return the liquor to the kettle and boil down to the consistency of tar, taking great care not to scorch or burn it. Then bottle close for use. Dose, 1 teaspoon 3 times a day until a cure is effected, using an herbal ointment, salve or oil on piles.

Apply burdock leaves all around the parts and back.

Chickweed chopped and boiled in lard, makes a fine cooling ointment.

Apply fresh juice of aloe vera.

Take excrescences which form upon the leaves of sumach, very finely powdered, an ounce; fresh lard, 6 ounces. Blend them together thoroughly. This is beneficial in piles, and often affords surprising relief. It may be confined to the parts by means of a bandage and a piece of lint or folded rag.

Boil about ½ ounce of smartweed root with 2 ounces of lard, and apply to piles 3 or 4 times a day. It may help ease pain and itching.

Hemorrhoids, internal and external. Drink 2 small whiskeyglassfuls of the fresh juice of mountain ash berries, 3 times daily for a considerable time. It will open the internal hemorrhoids and act as a laxative.

Make a strong decoction of chamomile flowers and use as a sitz bath, apply vaseline after and press rectum back gently.

The root of Jamestown weed, made into a salve, and the fundament greased with it, will afford speedy relief from pain.

When tumors become very painful, and are considerably inflamed, a poultice made of pulverized slippery elm bark and milk will be found to give great relief.

Add 1 ounce of white oak bark to 1 quart water; boil slowly till reduced to 1 pint, then strain. When cold use this liquid to bathe the piles. Apply with absorbent cotton. Relief is almost instantaneous.

W. H. Daley

Steep Solomon's seal root in a pint of milk for 3 nights. Bathe piles with the strained liquid.

L. Rowland, 1950

For protruding piles use the top side of fresh leaves of Adam's flannel or mullein for toilet paper at stool time and give the piles a good rubbing with the velvety leaves.

Use fresh dog-fennel leaves for wiping the piles.

Protruding and bleeding piles: put a generous portion of pilewort in a wide-mouthed bottle, add to it ½ pint raw linseed oil. Place it in a vessel of warm water and let steep for several hours. When cool apply as an ointment during the day 3 or 4 times or whenever convenient and upon retiring.

Make a salve of equal parts of shepherd's purse herb, stone root and pilewort in enough (unsalted) lard. Simmer until virtues are removed from botanicals. Stronger salve may be made by straining off the botanicals and adding fresh botanicals to the lard and repeating the process.

J. Vasil, 1950

For obstinate piles, blind, bleeding or otherwise, fresh poke berries are a sure cure. The berries ripen in September and remain until January. Press out the juice. Bathe the parts and inject with a syringe, or wet a soft cloth and press against the parts. Have known 3 injections to cure cases of many years' standing. It is harmless. In order to keep poke berry juice on hand steep berries in glycerine.

Take 1 ounce of poke root, and 1 ounce of burdock root, put them into a pint of boiling water, and let it steep awhile; when cool, add a little gin to prevent its souring, bottle it tight, and take from 2 to 4 tablespoons daily; or simmer sunflower seeds in cream and make it into an ointment; rub this ointment on the inside and outside, and for an injection use strong Castile soap suds.

Dr. A. A. Benezet, 1826

Piles bleeding: Make a strong decoction of yarrow herb, and drink freely; or, take a piece of poke root about the size of a hen's egg, put it into a pint of boiling water, and let it steep a few hours. When cool, take from 1 to 3 tablespoons, as the stomach will bear daily, before eating.

A strong decoction of yarrow herb has long been used as an external application for bleeding piles.

Take ½ ounce of bistort root, and alum root, simmer in 2 ounces of lard and 2 ounces mutton suet. Strain and add 1 ounce of olive oil. Mix well. Apply.

Make a salve by boiling the fresh leaves of celandine in lard. If accompanied by hemorrhage, add equal parts of shepherd's purse herb, knot grass herb, nettles herb, and witch hazel leaves.

If the parts are very sore or irritable, an injection is good, which may consist of an infusion of raspberry leaves, witch hazel leaves or sumach leaves, rendered somewhat mucilaginous with slippery elm bark. The liquid should always be strained, or the sediment will tend to aggravate the complaint.

Mrs. E. A. Howland, 1847

Take sweet elder, the inner bark, and simmer it in sweet cream, take the juice of camomile pounded and pressed out, and mix a tablespoon of this with a gill of the above, and use it night and morning constantly. This perhaps is as good a remedy as can be made externally for that troublesome disorder.

If outward, make an ointment of the leaves of burdock, sage, garden parsley and camomile; simmer them in a hog's lard or fresh butter and sweet oil; anoint the parts with it; drink ½ a gill of tar water 3 times a day; but if they are inward, drink essence of fir every night and tar water twice a day; a small ½ glass of this followed up for a month or 2 will effect a cure.

Take of mullein leaves and tobacco a handful, each; lard 1 pound; boil till all the strength is extracted, then press out and strain the lard, to which add 2 tablespoonfuls of powdered alum.

Another very excellent preparation for piles, whether blind or bleeding, is made of pumpkin seed oil, oil of fireweed, oil of horsemint, and linseed oil, equal parts; mix. To be rubbed upon the parts twice a day, and a piece of lint or cotton anointed with it, and worn over the fundament.

An ointment made of the bruised leaves of fireweed, simmered in fresh butter, relieves the hemorrhoids or piles.

Make a salve with equal parts of bittersweet root, mullein flowers and powdered slippery elm bark in enough sweet butter to thoroughly mix ingredients. Simmer under very low fire until virtues of botanicals are thoroughly incorporated in the butter. Use salve frequently.

N. J. R.

Take elder roots, hearts of plantain, of burdock roots, of mullein herb, mallows, catnip herb, and motherwort herb, a handful of each; to be stewed in 1 pound fresh butter—with this the patient is frequently to grease himself.

P. Smith, 1812

PLASTERS

Make a mixture of 1 part of mustard powder to 4 parts flour, for an adult, and 6 or 7 parts of flour if for a child. Stir the mixture into a thin paste with warm water and spread it thinly on a piece of cloth or brown paper, and cover with a thin cloth. Do not use boiling water in making the plaster. Oatmeal, bran, Indian meal, or flaxseed may be used instead of the flour.

Mix dry mustard with the white of an egg, or glycerine. This will avoid blistering.

When making mustard plasters, ground ginger and mustard are used in equal quantities, and if diluted with about ¼ the quantity of flour, the plaster will not blister. The ginger is better for all colds of a grippe nature. If mustard plasters are mixed with hot water, they act quicker.

Mix together 1 ounce each of powdered cloves, ground cinnamon and ground allspice, 2 ounces ground pepper and 3 or 4 ounces flour. Mix to a paste with a very little water and spread on muslin. If a more powerful plaster is required, substitute cayenne for black pepper.

Take a pitch pine knot and boil it in water, till all the gum is out. Then let it cool, and take off the pitch. Spread a plaster of this, and wear it on the side or breast, or wherever it may be wanted. If it is too powerful, temper it with a little rosin or beeswax.

Take pine tar and hemlock tree gum equal parts; stir in a teaspoon of sulphur: it is fit for use.

PLEURISY

Parched salt put in cloth and laid hot on pain will temporarily stop pleurisy.

Letter, 1931

197

Apply hot fomentation made with hops, wormwood, smartweed or catnip. Apply frequently and always hot to the affected side. Do not get night clothes or covers wet.

Rub the side with camphorated oil and cover over with a cotton jacket.

Pleurisy root is highly extolled for the cure of pleurisy. Boil 1 ounce of the root in 1½ pints of water for 10 minutes. Strain. Dose, a wine-glassful 2 or 3 times a day.

Gipsy recipe

POISON IVY, POISON OAK, etc.

Frequent bathing of the affected parts in water as hot as can be borne. If used immediately after exposure, it may prevent the eruption appearing. If later, it allays the itching, and gradually dries up the swellings, though they are very stubborn after they have once appeared. But an application every few hours keeps down the intolerable itching. In addition to this, the ordinary astringent ointments are useful.

Add 1 ounce of glycerin and 1 tablespoon carbolic acid to 1 pint of boiling water and use as a wash on affected parts.

Powdered chalk wet to a paste with water and applied thickly will give swift relief and prevent further inflammation in early stages.

Take a handful of quicklime, dissolve it in water, let it stand ½ hour, and then paint the poisoned parts with it. Three or 4 applications, generally cures.

Apply a wash made with 1 drachm calomel to 1 pint lime water.

Bicarbonate of soda applied in early stages, will often check ivy poisoning.

Bathe parts affected 2 or 3 times a day with sweet spirits of niter.

Make a strong solution of alum water and bathe the affected parts freely a few times, and it will effect a cure.

Dissolve 1 ounce of gum shellac in 6 ounces of sulphuric ether; cork tightly in a bottle; bathe the surface where the irritation appears with cold water and wipe dry; then apply the above solution; the ether will evaporate, leaving an elastic coating of gum, impervious to the air; in a few minutes the most distressing case of poison oak can be relieved; as the coating peels off, use more of the solution and the cure is effected in 24 hours.

A strong lye made of wood ashes gives instant relief. The dry ashes may be applied with equal good results.

A few drops of kerosene oil, rubbed in with the point of the finger or a piece of sponge, is a certain and speedy cure for the effects of the poison oak. Repeat for 3 or 4 days.

Olive oil is said to be a cure. In severe cases it is to be taken inwardly as well as applied externally. Dose: 2 tablespoonfuls 3 times a day, keeping the affected parts well oiled all the time. Anointing exposed parts with the oil will prevent poisoning.

Oil of goldenrod [*Solidago odora*] is never known to fail to cure poison from ivy, oak or sumac. If the skin be broken, put a little sweet oil with the oil of goldenrod.

Heavily salted milk applied to the parts affected by ivy poisoning and allowed to dry on, is said to be a very effective remedy for ivy poisoning.

May I tell you that mouse-ear herb boiled in milk cures the worst case of poison ivy in almost 24 hours and 3 days at the most. I had a young lady who was sitting on bath towels absolutely naked for 3 days. Her doctor wanted to take her to the hospital. After 1 treatment with mouse-ear she slept well all night. She had poison ivy over most of her body.

Take fresh green leaves of nightshade, mash up in fresh cream until cream turns green. Apply as poultice.

Take some good rich buttermilk in which you have beaten some green tansy leaves until the milk is thoroughly tinctured. Bathe the parts often (indeed, you could not do it too often) until relieved. Wet a cloth with the mixture at night, and lay it on, wetting as often as it feels dry.

The fresh leaves of jewel weed applied to poison ivy blisters will dry them up in 24 hours if applied frequently.

The bruised leaves of fireweed rubbed on the parts poisoned with ivy, give relief, if applied immediately after the first symptoms are perceived.

The common wild Indian turnip, or jack-in-the-pulpit is an excellent remedy when scraped and applied to the poisoned part. When the blisters have flattened, apply cold cream to heal them sooner.

The fresh green leaves of catnip herb rubbed on affected parts until the juice runs, is most efficacious no matter how advanced the case may be.

A strong decoction of sweet fern leaves was used as a wash for muskrat or wild parsnip poisoning.

For manchineel poisoning: bathe parts in sea water.

Slaves brought from the West Indies made poultices of the mashed leaves of pink trumpet tree [*Tabebuia heterophylla*] for manchineel poisoning. The leaves were also rubbed on the skin when one came in contact with a Portuguese-man-of-war.

Other botanicals that have been used in strong decoctions as washes for plant poisoning: gum plant [*Grindelia squarrosa*], dark-leaved mugwort [*Artemisia ludoviciana*], leaves and small branches of tag alder [*Alnus rubra*], witch hazel leaves and twigs [*Hamamelis virginiana*], horsetail grass [*Equisetum hyemale* or *E. arvense*], white or red oak bark [*Quercus alba* or *Q. rubra*], lobelia herb [*Lobelia inflata*], vervain herb [*Verbena hastata*], marsh rosemary [*Limonium carolinianum*] and numerous others. Most recipes recommend that the wash be applied as hot as can be borne.

POULTICES

Poultices should be applied as hot as can be borne, and frequently changed—the old poultice not being removed before the new one is at hand to replace it.

When applying poultice put wax paper between it and bandage so that the medical parts will not be absorbed by the bandage.

Poultices may be worn with more comfort, and removed with more ease, if the surface is spread over, before applying, with a little perfectly fresh lard or sweet oil.

Make a thick paste with ground flaxseed and scalding hot water. Spread paste about an inch thick upon a piece of thick muslin or linen and put over it a piece of thin cloth, which will serve to keep flaxseed from sticking to the skin. Apply poultice while it is hot and keep it warm by covering thickly with flannel. A poultice should be changed every 2 hours, the fresh poultice being ready to apply before the old one is removed.

Oatmeal poultices are more stimulating, and draw more rapidly than those made of flaxseed.

Mrs. A. Matteson, 1894

A bread poultice is made like the flaxseed, using stale bread crumbs instead of flaxseed.

A bread and milk poultice is made by substituting milk for water.

Charcoal poultices are made by adding ½ ounce of charcoal to a flaxseed poultice and by sprinkling a little of the charcoal over the poultice mixture.

The roots of garden carrots scraped and wilted, are good made into a poultice, to subdue inflammation and swelling, and heal old sores.

Take of boiled carrots, bruised 1 pound; flour, 1 ounce; butter, ½ ounce. Mix them with as much warm water as to form a pulp. This will be found a valuable application to ulcerated sores and swellings, scrofulous sores of the irritable kind, and many other inveterate ulcers.

The leaves of garden horseradish are a good application, however they are much more powerful than other leaves and generally blister on tender skin.

Ground ginger used for plasters or poultices instead of mustard, is just as good to draw and it never blisters.

Ginger is used as a substitute for mustard poultice, but if the patient has very delicate skin, it is better to prepare the poultice of crushed flaxseed and then sprinkle it thickly with powdered ginger.

Take ½ cup of flour and 1 teaspoon of each kind of ground spice available, wet with alcohol or whiskey. This poultice may be left on any length of time without blistering.

A writer gives an instance in which a woman's arm was swelled to an enormous size and painfully inflamed. A poultice was made of stewed pumpkins, which was renewed every 15 minutes, and in a short time produced a perfect cure. The fever drawn out by the poultices made them extremely offensive as they were taken off.

Miss T. S. Shute, 1878

The leaves of common grape vine boiled with barley meal makes a cooling poultice for inflammations and wounds.

Mrs. A. Matteson, 1894

The leaves of peach tree make a good poultice. Boil and add a little meal and a pinch of salt. Place on soft cloth and apply hot. Change when cool.

Mrs. M. H., 1960

Catnip herb made into a poultice is soothing for external inflammation and especially for boils. Fresh or dried catnip is also used with bread poultices.

Pour boiling water over a handful of hops and set them aside to steep for several minutes. Then squeeze through a strainer and spread hops upon a cloth.

A poultice made of pounded fresh horsetail grass has remarkable properties according to an informant.

The whole plant of comfrey beaten to a cataplasm, and applied hot as a poultice, has always been deemed excellent for soothing pain in any tender, inflamed or suppurating part.

Outward inflammations of all kinds yield to poultices made with common violet herb.

The leaves and pith of mullein make a valuable poultice for sprains, white swelling and inflammations.

The fresh leaves of mullein, wet with vinegar, are good to apply externally where there is pain, swellings, or inflammation.

A poultice of the green leaves of jimson weed, or if dry, softened with warm water, is an admirable application to the bowels, or abdomen, in inflammation of the stomach or bowels.

Fenugreek seed is the best of all remedies for dissolving tumors that I know of. It works slowly, painlessly, but lastingly and thoroughly. It is applied in a manner similar to flaxseed; the powder mixed with water is boiled to a paste, and put on the suffering part in linen rags.

German recipe

Wormwood herb pounded with spirits is good to put on bruises; also united with double tansy and hops pounded together and wet with spirits or vinegar, it is excellent to apply to any external inflammation, or a pain in the side; if you have not the 3 articles above named use what you have.

P. E. Sanborn, 1836

Make a very strong tea of white oak bark, and thicken with corn meal to the consistence of a poultice; apply it as hot as can be borne, and change it every 2 hours. This will disperse tumors.

Take of mayweed or the flowers, a suitable quantity, bruise to a soft pulp, and boil for a short time in a small quantity of water; then stir in corn meal until of a suitable consistence for a poultice, spread on thick cloth and apply to the neck, renewing when it becomes dry. This is recommended as being highly useful for the sore throat of scarlet fever, and for all swellings and inflammations.

Smartweed is a powerful antiseptic, and allays inflammation, discusses [disperses] cold swellings, particularly such as affect the knee joint, and dissolves congealed blood in bruises, blows, etc. For these purposes, it should be applied in a strong decoction and poultice. To remove inflammation or to prevent or check mortification, take the herb, bruise and boil it in a suitable quantity of water; bathe the part affected with the liquor, and apply the buised herb hot, as a fomentation, renewing as it becomes cold.

H. Howard, 1857

A decoction of fresh chicory roots is used as a poultice for inflammation and ulcers. Boiled roots are not strained off.

Bad ulcers and hard tumors have been removed by the application of the bruised root of yellow dock in poultice.

The fresh root of poke roasted in hot ashes until soft, and mashed and made into a poultice, is an excellent application for tumors, felons, and the like, to scatter them, or prevent them from coming to a head; or, if too late for that, to hasten suppuration.

Take of the bark of the roots of the common sumach, any quantity; bruise it well, and boil in sweet milk, catnip tea, or water, for 20 minutes; then thicken with corn meal or crackers to a proper consistence for a poultice. This is a highly valuable poultice for all kinds of foul ulcers, and especially those which affect the bones.

The fresh root of common cat tail flag, bruised and wet with cold water, and applied to external inflammations, gives great relief. It may be applied to sore eyes, or any hot humor, swelling, etc.

Dr. D. Rogers, 1824

The Indians use a decoction of the roots of nine bark for fomenting and poulticing, in all cases which require such applications. It removes the anguish, and cures a burn beyond credibility; cases verging on mortification, felons, swellings, rising of a woman's breast, etc. yield to its application beyond anything else. To apply it, boil the roots and make a strong decoction, then take of the liquor and thicken up a poultice with bran or Indian meal, this may be put into a little bag made of a thin cloth, and apply it as warm and as moist as will be agreeable; this may be repeated as often as you will, until the pain or inflammation is quite gone, or the wound or sore cured. Linen or cotton cloths dipt in the liquor, hot, and applied as warm as can be borne, and then kept close while the case remains, and so repeated, will be a good way to apply it.

P. Smith, 1812

The elm is an excellent thing for a poultice, as it is very soft and healing. It is good to mix it with pounded cracker, to make a poultice, as it keeps the poultice soft.

Take of yeast, a sufficient quantity, and thicken it to the proper consistence with charcoal and slippery elm bark finely pulverized. This is highly useful applied to ulcers in a gangrenous or mortified condition.

Take the bark of the root of sassafras, bruise it well and boil in sweet milk or water, when it may be thickened to a proper consistence with meal, slippery elm, or flaxseed. This is also a valuable application for mortified ulcers.

Mix powdered slippery elm bark with hot water or with hot water and milk to make a smooth paste. Spread paste on clean cloth, bandage and apply over the parts affected. In cases of abscesses and old wounds, the slippery elm paste should be spread between cloths. If applied to parts of the body where there is hair, the face of the poultice should be smeared with olive oil before applying. Beach wrote that this poultice exceeds every other in point of efficacy. It is of almost universal application, and removes inflammation sooner than any other.

Boil 1 ounce of dried wormwood herb in 1 pint of water for 10 or 15 minutes. Strain off herb and use enough of the wormwood decoction to make a paste with powdered slippery elm bark that has previously been mixed with finely powdered charcoal (equal parts of each). Apply paste to bandage. Renew bandage and paste 3 or more times per day.

Take of lobelia and slippery elm, each in powder, 1 ounce; weak lye, hot, a sufficient quantity to form a poultice; mix. This is a useful poultice in fistula, wounds, whitlow, boils, erysipelatous inflammations, stings by insects, and external inflammations, swellings, etc., accompanied with pain.

Other botanicals used in poultices: fresh mashed leaf blades of sea onion or squills, fresh mashed leaves of cabbage—preferably the blue or so-called red cabbage, bruised leaves of houseleek or hens-and-chickens, fresh leaves of common or ribwort plantain, fresh marsh-mallow leaves, marigold leaves, shepherd's purse herb, mashed leaves of burdock, tamarind pulp, and many other non-toxic parts of plants.

PREGNANCY

TO FACILITATE CHILDBIRTH

The blueberry root [*Caulophyllum thalictroides*] is said to be the great medicine that the squaws use at the birth of their children. Experience has however proved, among white women, that its assistance is very special. It is to be made use of in the following manner—Take a good handful of green or dry roots, make it into a tea (say ½ pint) give the ½ of it, and fill up with hot water; repeat drinking every 10 minutes, or oftener, until it has its effect.

When a woman finds that she is taken in labor, let her drink as above, having her help at hand—if it is not her time, she will probably get easy and be well; but if it is her time, expect the delivery will be facilitated with much safety. It is to be noticed, that if the anguish attending the delivery is not moderated, the doses have not been strong enough; for they act on the same stimulant principles that opium does—and a suitable degree of indirect debility will moderate the great distress that must otherwise be experienced. The delivery is facilitated by it, so as seldom to be slow and lingering. But the great benefit is the state of safety and of speedy and sure recovery that the mother experiences afterwards.

The squaws, I have heard, drink a little of a tea of this root for 2 or 3 weeks before their expected time. I have given this tea in a case of inflammation of the uterus, and found it a speedy cure.

The tea of this root is neither a purge nor a vomit, but acts as a stimulus to the nervous system, till by indirect debility it will give ease in any distress. I believe that it is always safe.

P. Smith, 1812

Squaw vine is an invaluable plant for child-bearing women. I first obtained the knowledge of its use from a tribe of Indians residing in the west part of New York, though not without considerable difficulty and intrigue. The squaws drank it in decoction for 2 or 3 weeks previous to, and during delivery, and it was the use of this herb that rendered that generally dreaded event, so remarkably safe and easy with them.

Elisha Smith, Physician and Surgeon, 1830

Black snake-root [Cimicifuga racemosa] is very serviceable in female complaints, whence the Indians call it squaw-root: it promotes menstrual discharge, and is peculiarly serviceable in removing pains and sickness of the stomach and heartburn in pregnant women. I have used it in such cases with astonishing good effect. The mode of administering it, is in a tea; take a handful, say 2 ounces, add a pint of boiling water, keep it where it will be warm, and drink occasionally 2 or 3 swallows at a time, through the day. It should be used in connexion with slippery elm, before childbirth, as it generally assists nature in such cases.

P. E. Sanborn, 1836

Take 2 ounces each of cramp bark, blue cohosh, slippery elm, raspberry leaves, squaw vine, orange peel and bitterroot [*Gentiana catesbaei*]. Simmer gently in sufficient water to keep the herbs covered, for 2 hours, strain, and simmer gently down to 1 quart, let it stand to cool, then add 1 cup of granulated sugar, and 4 ounces of alcohol. Dose, a tablespoon 2 or 3 times a day, for several weeks before birth of child and as needed after birth.

Mrs. A. Matteson, 1894

A tea made of the leaves of red raspberry, sweetened, with milk in it, is very pleasant, and may be used freely. It is the best thing for women in travail, of any article I know of. Give a strong tea of it, with a little cayenne, sweetened, and it will regulate everything as nature requires. If the pains are untimely, it will make all quiet; if timely and lingering, give more cayenne and yellow lady slipper root tea. When the child is born, give it some of the tea with sugar and milk in it; this prevents sore mouth; and the tea is good to wash sore nipples with.

S. Thomson, 1831

An infusion of slippery elm bark is an excellent thing for women to take for a month or 6 weeks before the birth of children, as it makes the birth of the child much more easy and safe than without it.

Elias Smith, Physician, 1826

From the time movement of the baby is felt, till time of the birth drink 1 cup of the following each day: Steep 1 or 2 teaspoons of the root of spikenard in a cup of boiling water for 10 to 15 minutes. When cool, strain and drink cold.

Indian recipe

An infusion made of feverfew herb makes a good drink for mothers before and after confinement.

TO PREVENT ABORTION OR MISCARRIAGE

The bark of the root of *Viburnum prunifolium* appears to exert an especial tonic influence upon the uterus, and is highly recommended in cases of threatened abortion and as a preventive in cases of habitual miscarriage.

J. King, M.D., 1855

A decoction of star root taken in small doses 3 or 4 times a day is said to be an almost infallible remedy to prevent abortion.

A mild tea of common garden sage is a good drink in time of pregnancy for those who are liable to abortion.

NAUSEA OR SICK STOMACH

Drink a tea made by steeping 2 tablespoons of ordinary oats in a pint of boiling water for ½ hour.

In some cases lemon or lime juice or a little vinegar in water gives relief.

Of columbo root and chamomile flowers make a strong tea, in which you may add a little ginger. Let this tea get cold, and give 3 or 4 tablespoons occasionally. Or you may obtain columbo root in powder, and give 15 or 20 grains, mixed with a few drops of peppermint, and a little good old spirits of any kind. Or take an ounce of columbo root, and bruise it with a hammer; then pour a pint of boiling water on it, and let it get cold. Take a wine-glassful of this decoction, with a few drops of peppermint in it, 3 or 4 times a day, or when you feel sickness in the stomach. Where the vomiting or puking is very severe, apply the stewed leaves of garden mint to the pit of the stomach; the application must be warm. Ginger tea and mint tea are also good remedies.

J. C. Gunn, M.D., 1830

Squaws used a decoction made from the roots of Indian cup-plant to alleviate vomiting of pregnancy.

CONSTIPATION

If a laxative is needed drink a mild infusion of cascara sagrada. Steep 1 teaspoon of the bark in a cupful of hot water for 3 or 4 minutes. Drink ½ cup or full cup as needed. Drastic drugs must be avoided.

As a purgative American colombo is substituted to rhubarb in many cases, particularly for children and pregnant women, being found serviceable in the constipation of pregnancy. It has the advantage of not heating the body. Cold water is said to add to its efficiency and prevent nausea or emesis.

TO RELIEVE SCALDING AND ITCHING CAUSED BY URINE

Keep bowels gently open and drink frequently small doses of infusion of slippery elm bark, marshmallow root, or flaxseed. An infusion made of peach tree leaves or mullein herb are also recommended for acridity of urine.

S. Pancoast, M.D., 1901

CRAMPS

Cramp bark is very effective in relaxing cramps and spasms of all kinds, as asthma, hysteria, cramps of the limbs or other parts in females, especially during pregnancy, and it is said to be highly beneficial to those who are subject to convulsions during pregnancy, or at the time of parturition, preventing the attacks entirely, if used daily for the last 2 or 3 months of gestation.

J. King, M.D., 1855

CONVULSIONS

Tansy herb will stop convulsions in confinement. Take fresh herb, crush it and put it to the nose. It is also good to keep a woman from miscarriage. Make an infusion and drink it and make a little bag and put some in it and wear it under the arms.

Letter, 1931

SWELLING OF FEET AND LIMBS

Drink freely of infusions of queen-of-the-meadow root, haircap moss, or marshmallow root.

DISTENTION OF SKIN

When the skin of the belly becomes cracked and sore, as in the advanced months of pregnancy, much relief will be afforded by rubbing it frequently with warm olive oil, in which a small quantity of camphor has been dissolved.

AFTERPAINS

Apply warm fomentations to the belly made of hops, tansy or other bitter herbs in whiskey, use freely as tea an infusion made with avens root or blue cohosh root.

Few people perhaps are aware of the value of tansy, particularly in regulating flooding, after childbirth. From 1 to 2 tumblerfuls, of the strong tea of double tansy, and spirits, with molasses, may be taken in the course of 24 hours, for a number of days after the child is born. I know this to be good, having proved it. It regulates the flooding, whether it be too little or too much; it gives vigor and energy to the system.

P. E. Sanborn, 1836

One pill of camphor will relieve, or every 2 or 3 hours will relieve or entirely cure afterpains in parturient women.

DISCHARGES AFTER CHILDBIRTH

The roots of healall are used by the Indians chiefly for women's complaints. Use it in tea or decoctions, which may freely be drunk, being quite innocent, but very efficacious. It is a remedy for pains attending the peculiar state, or purgations of females; it may be given both before and after childbirth; it will restore obstructed lochia, and briefly speaking, it is the best women's root that I know.

P. Smith, 1812

Take 4 parts eryngo root [*Eryngium aquaticum*], 2 parts kava kava root [*Piper methysticum*], 3 parts palmetto berries [*Serenoa serrulata*], 2 parts thuja leaves [*Thuja occidentalis*], 4 parts shepherd's purse [*Capsella bursa-pastoris*], and 4 parts parsley piert herb [*Alchemilla arvensis*]. Mix well. Boil ½ ounce of the mixture in 1 pint of water for 5 minutes. Strain when cool. Drink in small doses 3 times a day between meals.

Drink an infusion in small doses 3 or 4 times a day made with equal parts of *Ephedra americana* sticks, *Larrea divaricata* leaves, and *Anemopsis californica* roots.

RHEUMATISM

Celery, raw, stewed, or in soup is the cure par excellence for rheumatism, and very simple and agreeable.

Take 3 ounces celery seed, 2 ounces chamomile flowers, put in 2 quarts of water, and simmer down to 3 pints. Strain and bottle and keep in a cool place. Dose, 1 wineglassful before each meal.

Make a sirup of fresh horseradish roots by boiling them in water and sufficient sugar to make it palatable. Dose, 2 or 3 teaspoons 2 or 3 times a day.

Take the bark of a bearing crabapple tree, put a sufficient amount of it into good whiskey, making it very strong. Drink a wineglass of this 3 times daily until a gallon has been used or until results.

K. R. R.

The bark of wild black cherry tree dried and made into a drink is good.

Fill a mason jar ⅛ full of fresh [washed] dandelion roots. Pour over this again as much good whiskey and allow it to stand for 10 days. Take teaspoon every morning. The dandelion root must have the white milk for best results.

L. Foerster, 1920

Boil 1 ounce dandelion root in 1½ pints of water for 20 minutes. Strain. Dose: a wineglass twice daily.

Steep ½ ounce each of dandelion root, Virginia snakeroot, burdock root in 1 quart of Holland gin. Dose, 2 tablespoons before breakfast.

Mix the following powdered ingredients: 1 ounce dandelion root, ½ ounce poke root, 1 ounce mayapple root, 1 ounce rhubarb root. Put into "oo" capsules and take 1 each night and morning, in spring and fall.

Take 1 pint of poke berries (equals 1 pound), 1 pound of brown sugar, ½ gallon of whiskey. Steep ingredients overnight. Dose: 1 tablespoon 3 times a day.

Mrs. W. H. M., 1954

Steep 1 pint of poke berries, and 1 tablespoon of sulphur in 1 quart of alcohol or brandy. Allow to stand 24 hours. Dose, 1 tablespoon 3 times a day.

Make a decoction of poke root and take 4 swallows a day for 3 weeks.

Take 2 pints of best rye whiskey, add ½ pound ground burdock seed and ½ pint poke berry juice. Mix and shake well. Dose, for adults, 1½ or 2 tablespoons night and morning.

Coffee made from the green berry [*Coffea arabica*] will bring relief, if it does not effect a permanent cure. To a teacup of cold water add a tablespoon of green coffee. Allow it to steep over-night, and drink before breakfast in the morning.

Drink an infusion made with the dried leaves of sweet fern 3 times a day.

Chew the root of angelica and swallow the juice several times during the day.

Drink a tea made of rosemary leaves before going to bed and as hot as possible, and another cupful in the morning before breakfast.

Steep 1 teaspoon of queen-of-the-meadow root in 1 cup of boiling water and allow to stand 20 minutes. Drink 1 or 2 cupfuls a day. May be taken in small draughts.

Cocash root removes obstructions of the fluids. The root, bruised and steeped in brandy or other spirits, and taken frequently, relieves such as are afflicted with rheumatic complaints.

Drink 3 times a day a tea made of horsemint herb.

Mix together ¼ teaspoon red pepper, 1 teaspoon sulphur and 2 teaspoons molasses. Take this as a dose every morning for a week, then skip a week, then take it for another week, and you will experience great relief.

Steep 1 tablespoon of powdered watermelon seeds in 1 cup of boiling water. Drink 2 or 3 times a day.

Mrs. M. G., 1950

Steep 1 tablespoon yerba del pasmo in 1 cup of boiling water for 5 to 10 minutes. Drink 2 or 3 times a day.

Mrs. S. Smith

Gobernadora or creosote bush was much used by the Indians, Mexicans and people of Spanish ancestry in the southwestern states for rheumatism. The tea was made of the leaves.

Mix equal parts of Oregon grape root with gobernadora leaves. Steep 1 teaspoon of the mixture in 1 cup of boiling water for 5 to 10 minutes. Strain and take ½ cupful at a time twice a day.

F. A., 1948

Take 2 parts of gobernadora, 1 part black cohosh, 1 part poke root. Mix. Steep 1 teaspoon in 1 cup of boiling water for 20 minutes. Take ½ cupful twice a day.

Mrs. J. S., 1950

Steep 1 teaspoon of black cohosh in 1 cup of boiling water. Allow to steep 20 minutes and strain. Drink wineglassful 3 times a day.

Take equal parts of black cohosh root, blue cohosh root, poke root, yellow dock root, blue flag root, prickly ash root, burdock root, and dandelion root, mix well. Boil 2 tablespoons in a pint of water for 5 minutes. When cool, strain and drink freely. Avoid rich and spicy foods.

Take of dried rattleroot ½ ounce; gum guaiacum ½ ounce; juice of poke berries 1½ gills; French brandy 1 quart. Mix. Shake it frequently for 2 or 3 days, when it will be fit for use. Drink of this as often as can be borne without producing intoxication, until a cure is effected.

Tincture of gum guaiacum, 10 to 15 drops, 3 times a day. I have never known it to fail making a cure, except in cases of long standing, when it will afford great relief.

Steep 1 ounce gum guaiacum in 1 pint of best brandy. Dose, take as much as you can bear, and take it clear. Repeat the dose until a cure is effected.

Take 1 ounce of gum guaiacum, ½ ounce of gum myrrh, and 2 drachms of niter; put into 1 quart best gin. Take 1 tablespoon in cold water morning, noon and night.

Steep 2 ounces Rochelle salts, 2 ounces of guaiacum, ¼ pound hemlock tree bark [*Tsuga canadensis*] in 1 quart of best brandy. Dose 1 tablespoon 3 times a day.

M.H., 1951

One ounce each of sulphur and cream of tartar, ½ ounce rhubarb, 1 teaspoon guaiacum and 16 ounces of honey. Take 1 tablespoon of this night and morning in a glass of lemonade or water.

Take 1 part each of guaiacum, cascara bark, hawthorn berries, 1½ parts red clover flowers, quaking aspen bark, and 2 parts yarrow herb and uva ursi leaves. Place ½ ounce of this mixture in 1 pint of water and simmer slowly for 20 minutes. Strain when cool. Dose, 2 tablespoons after each meal.

Make a strong decoction of sarsaparilla [*Smilax officinale*] and water by boiling. To 1 quart of sarsaparilla decoction add 10 teaspoons sassafras bark of root, 10 teaspoons guaiacum shavings, 10 teaspoons licorice root, and 3 teaspoons of mezereon bark [*Dirca palustris*]. Boil 15 minutes and strain when cool. Dose, a wineglassful twice a day.

Take 3 ounces each of tinctures sarsaparilla and quassia, 1 ounce iodide potash, 20 grains quinine, 1 pint of water. Put all into a quart bottle, and shake when taking. Dose 1 tablespoon just before each meal.

Mrs. M. W. Ellsworth, 1897

Finest Turkey rhubarb, ½ ounce; carbonate magnesia, 1 ounce; mix intimately; keep well corked in glass bottle. Dose, 1 teaspoon, in milk and sugar, the first thing in the morning; repeat till cured.

Miss E. Neill, 1890

Take equal parts of linden flowers, queen-of-the-meadow root, wild carrot seed, hair-cap moss, buchu leaves and saffron, mix thoroughly. Place 8 teaspoons in a pan with 2 cups of boiling water. Allow to steep for ½ hour or more, then strain. Take ½ glass in morning and ½ glass at night. Keep bowels free.

R. H., 1950

Take ½ ounce gentian root and ½ ounce bittersweet root, and 1 ounce each of the following, tag alder, princess pine leaves, colombo root, yarrow herb and mayapple root. Soak mixture 48 hours in 1 quart best Holland gin, then strain. Dose, 1 tablespoon before each meal. If this physics too much decrease dose.

Take 1 ounce of seneca snakeroot, 2 ounces white pine bark, 2 ounces burdock seeds. Mix thoroughly. Steep 1 teaspoon of this mixture in 1 cup of boiling water. Drink ½ cupful at a time several times a day.

Take of Virginia snakeroot 1 ounce; white pine bark 2 ounces; burdock seeds 2 ounces; prickly ash 2 ounces. Pulverize all together, and add a gallon of water; boil to 3 pints. Take ½ pint a day divided into 2 or 3 doses. An excellent decoction in chronic cases.

W. Beach, M.D., 1833

Many physicians place great reliance on bark of prickly ash for its power in rheumatic complaints. The bark is most frequently given in decoction, an ounce being boiled in about a quart of water. About a pint taken in the course of a day, diluted with water sufficient to render it palatable by lessening the pungency. It was warm and grateful to the stomach, produced no nausea nor effect upon the bowels, and excited little, if any, perspiration. I have given the powdered bark in doses of 10 and 20 grains with considerable benefit. In 1 case it effectually removed the complaint in a few days. I have known it, however to fail entirely in obstinate cases.

J. Bigelow, M.D., 1820

Put the following ingredients in 2 quarts of boiling water: 1 ounce mayapple root, 1 ounce dandelion root, 1 ounce burdock root, 1 ounce yellow dock root, 2 ounces prickly ash bark, 1 ounce marshmallow root, ½ ounce Turkey rhubarb, 1 ounce gentian root, 1 ounce chamomile flowers, 1 ounce red clover flowers. Simmer under low fire for 6 hours. Strain and add ½ pint of best gin. Take ½ whiskey glass 3 times a day.

Dr. Gifford, 1912

Take of poke root, blue flag root, prickly ash, black cohosh root, bitter root, each, in powder, 1 ounce, whisky 2 quarts; mix. Let it stand for 10 or 12 days, frequently shaking. Dose, 1 tablespoon 2 or 3 times a day, in a glass of sweetened water.

Take of white pine, poke root, black cohosh, sassafras bark of root, sulphur, each, in coarse powder, 1 ounce; whiskey 2 pints; mix. Prepare and use in the same manner as the preceding.

J. King, M.D., 1864

Take of blue flag root, prickly ash, sweet flag root, bloodroot, each 4 ounces; powder and steep in brandy. Dose, from 1 tablespoon to a wineglassful 3 times a day.

Take a handful of blue flag root, put it into a pint of spirits, and let it stand a few days. Take a teaspoon 3 times a day to begin with, and increase by degrees to a tablespoon 3 times a day.

INTERNAL AND EXTERNAL MEDICATION

Take a handful of rheumatism-weed, a handful of horseradish roots, elecampane roots, prickly ash, bittersweet root, wild cherry bark, mustard seed, and a pint of tar water; put into 2 quarts of brandy. Drink a small glassful every morning, noon and night, before eating. Bathe the part affected with salt and rum, by a warm fire.

Take a single handful of sassafras bark of root, 1 ounce of gum camphor, 1 ounce of grated ginger root, and 1 quart of best brandy. Let the whole be steeped moderately 8 to 10 hours. For a dose, ⅓ of a wineglass, 3 or 4 times a day. Increase the dose if necessary. Bathe the part affected with the same, and use considerable friction with a red flannel, as hard as you can bear it. This generally gives relief in a few days, by being careful about taking cold for a short time.

Rheumatism in the loins. Sit over hemlock boughs, and drink poke berries steeped in brandy, for 3 weeks every day. Only sit 3 times. Or shower with cold water and drink brandy all the time; or drink brandy and bathe the part affected, with salt and rum, hot as can be borne, by a fire. Repeat it 6 days.

Take a tablespoon of pitch from a white pine log, and same quantity of sulphur, and a spoonful of honey. Add these to 2 quarts of the best ¼ proof brandy, and shake till it is dissolved. Cork it up tight for use. Take a tablespoon 3 times a day, before eating, and bathe the part affected in salt, and some of the same brandy, as hot as you can bear it.

EXTERNAL APPLICATIONS AND METHODS USED TO PALLIATE PAINS OF RHEUMATISM

Keep the fur side of a cat hide against lower part of the back or let a live cat lay on the lap everytime you sit down. It was believed the cat would eventually acquire all the rheumatism from the patient.

Old German recipe

Heat a flat iron sufficiently to vaporize vinegar. Cover heated flat iron with woolen fabric, then moisten fabric with vinegar. Apply as hot as can be borne on painful spot. Repeat application 2 or 3 times a day.

A very simple remedy for rheumatism of the extremities, and one that very often gives great relief is, to take a large piece of thick flannel, sprinkle it well with finely pulverized sulphur, and then bind snugly about the limb, with the sulphur next to the skin.

Take 1 pint of cider vinegar, 1 pint of turpentine, 4 fresh eggs, put the shells and all in vinegar, let stand until the vinegar eats the eggs all up, then add the turpentine.

Use a small lump of alum, as big as a walnut. Pound it fine, and dissolve it in water; bathe the affected part every night and morning, and keep a piece in your pocket, and you will seldom, if ever, be troubled with this painful disorder. This looks rather too simple to be relied on, but it is one of the best remedies known, and comes well authenticated. We all know that red flannel is the best article that ever was worn for the disorder. It is the alum which is in the cloth which makes it preferable to any other color. [Old time dyers used alum as a mordant to set the color.]

P. F. Bowker, 1836

Soak cotton batting in alcohol and camphor and apply.

Take 1 pint of turpentine, 1 pint of vinegar and the whites of 12 eggs—this makes a creamy liniment. Camphor is a good addition.

Take 1 pint spirits of camphor, 1 pint coon, bear, or skunk oil and 1 pint spirits of turpentine. Shake before using and apply 3 times daily. Rub vigorously for 20 to 30 minutes.

Take 1 part olive oil, 2 parts spirits of camphor and ¼ part cayenne pepper. Shake well before using.

Take ½ ounce each of oils of hemlock tree and cedar, 1 ounce each of oils origanum and sassafras, 1 ounce of aqua ammonia and pulverized capsicum and ½ ounce each spirits of turpentine and gum camphor. Put these ingredients in a quart bottle and fill it with pure alcohol.

Bathe parts with tincture of cayenne pepper 1 ounce in a quart of alcohol. Apply warm with a piece of flannel. Parts may also be bathed 2 or 3 times a day with the following warm mixture: 1 ounce each of oil of sassafras, oil of hemlock, oil of red cedar, oil of spearmint, turpentine, olive oil, and camphor.

The oil obtained by distilling the shavings of red cedar, is a very valuable application for pains of rheumatism.

Cajeput or sassafras oils often afford immediate relief on anointing the affected part. Oils may be diluted with small portion of olive oil.

A good liniment is made of ½ pint spirits of turpentine, 1 pint vinegar, 10 drops oil of sassafras and the yolk of 1 egg.

Take equal parts of strong vinegar, sweet oil and turpentine, and put in a well corked bottle. Bathe the parts affected with rheumatism with hot water, wipe dry and then apply this liniment, rubbing it in well. Do this every night until relieved.

Take cucumbers, when full grown, and put them into a pot with a little salt; then put the pot over a slow fire, where it should remain for about 1 hour; then take the cucumbers and press them, the juice from which must be put into bottles, corked up tight, and placed in the cellar, where they should remain for about a week; then wet a flannel rag with the liquid, and apply it to the parts affected.

A strong decoction used as a wash, or the wilted leaves used as a poultice of yerba mansa was believed to be an infallible cure for rheumatism.

Red pepper, infused in spirits, makes an excellent wash in rheumatism.

The rheumatism may often be effectually cured by bathing the part affected with decoctions of ground hemlock [*Taxus minor*].

Take a large handful of smart weed, bruise it and add as much sharp vinegar as it will absorb; warm it in a pot, or pan, and lay it on the part affected as a fomentation, or poultice, and renew it frequently. If it should prove too painful, as it sometimes will when applied to tender skin, mix it with cornmush or bran.

SCIATIC RHEUMATISM

Many years ago, a farm laborer was troubled with sciatic rheumatism. An old man showed the laborer a plant that could cure his condition. After taking an infusion made with the plant for some time, he was entirely relieved. The laborer offered his secret to this writer for $5,000.00; later for $3,000.00, and so on until the price was $2.00. After paying for the secret, the writer was given a few broken stems, leaves and 1 seed. The seed was the key to the identity—the plant was common bugleweed [*Lycopus virginicus*].

Drink 2 or 3 times a day a wineglassful of a decoction made of the roots of black cohosh.

Infuse 1 ounce of the herb ragwort in 1 pint of water as if making tea. Strain and take a wineglassful 3 times a day.

Take 1 gallon jar of green thistle leaves, commonly called bull thistle. After the jar is filled with the green leaves pour in all the water you can. Put over stove in granite-iron kettle or pan and boil down to ½ the quantity of water. Strain and place it where it will keep cold. Drink a wineglassful before each meal. Also make a weak tea of sweet flag or chew some sweet flag root 3 times a day. A sure cure. Repeat if necessary. Equally as good for neuralgia.

E. Boyle, 1916

RINGWORM

Most cases are cured simply by scratching around the outer surface with the point of a sharp pin. The disease will not pass the line, if the skin be thus cut.

A very simple, yet effective, manner of curing ringworm is to place on the affected part, for a short time every night, a copper coin which has remained for some time in vinegar, and is still wet with the liquid. It is also well to bathe the ringworm with a solution of 2 grains iodide of potash in 1 ounce water.

Make a paste of gunpowder and vinegar and apply.

Apply kerosene with finger several times a day.

Apply a poultice of sulphur and fresh butter.

Strong tobacco juice applied frequently is a certain cure.

Put some tobacco with some water, and boil it, and add some vinegar and strong lye to the liquor: wash the parts affected often.

Apply the juice of the rind of the black walnut.

Boil burdock root in vinegar and use as a wash to part affected.

Take bloodroot, slice it fine, and put it in vinegar; wash the parts affected with the liquid and it will cure.

Take yellow dock root, wash and cut in small pieces, simmer in vinegar, and when the strength is extracted, strain and apply the vinegar to the parts affected 3 times a day.

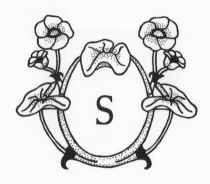

SCALL HEAD

The oil of skunk is good for scall head, and is used in making various kinds of ointments.

Take 1 pint of pine tar, and put it into a gallon of water; warm it well, and stir well together. Let it settle, and pour it off for use. With this wash the head of the child frequently, or shave off the hair, and let it wear a tarred cap. To cleanse the blood, take 1 peck of sarsaparilla roots, ½ peck of burdock roots and 1 handful of dog mackimus bark. Boil these together, and let the child drink freely of the liquor.

Take 2 ounces of raspberry leaves, and boil them in a quart of water for 20 minutes; pour the liquor boiling hot upon 1 ounce of lobelia, and bathe the head with this night and morning, but not twice in the same liquor, after which apply white ointment. (White ointment: Take 1 pound fresh butter, 1 ounce tincture iodine, 2 ounces oil origanum. Mix well together.) Keep the head covered during the day with a cap. As this disease results from a disordered state of the body, means must be taken to purify the blood and strengthen the system. Of the compound decoction of sarsaparilla give a tablespoon 4 times a day. If the disease commences in the spring, give a tablespoon of the expressed juice of clivers or nettles 3 times a day.

Boil the fresh root of Indian turnip in hog's lard to the consistence of an ointment.

SCROFULA

Drink an infusion made of the leaves or buds of black walnut.

Yellow dock root has proved very useful in scrofula. It is given in powder or decoction. Two ounces of the fresh root bruised, or 1 ounce of the dried, may be boiled in a pint of water, of which 2 fluid ounces may be given at a dose, and repeated as the stomach will bear.

A tea made of ripe, dried whortle berries, and drunk in place of water, is a sure and speedy cure for scrofula difficulties, however bad.

*The Modern Home Cook Book
and Family Physician,* about 1880

Take the roots of hellebore, pound and wet them with vinegar, and apply this poultice to the part affected. For a common drink, take equal quantities of wild lettuce and noble liverwort; infuse them in water, and let the patient drink freely.

Codfish skins applied to the part affected, will often cure.

Administer 1 drachm of Peruvian bark; ½ in the morning and ½ at night; also, give the patient 20 drops of the oil of tar, at 11 o'clock in the morning and at 4 o'clock in afternoon.

Take of powdered eggshells 1 teaspoon (or powdered oyster shells) mixed with Peruvian bark, ⅛ part, 2 or 3 times a day.

Give small portions of sulphur daily till cured.

SALVES FOR SCROFULOUS SKIN DISEASE

Make a salve of twinleaf root or deer's tongue stewed in lard.

Take a handful of elder bark put in a ½ gallon of water. Boil down to ½ pint, strain and in ½ pint of cream, simmer it slowly down to a salve. Apply daily.

SCURVY

A bath made of vinegar and water, in which the whole body can be frequently bathed, will be of essential service; as will also the plentiful use of ripe fruits; sauerkraut, or pickled cabbage is also an excellent remedy.

J. C. Gunn, M.D., 1830

Dissolve 3 ounces of common saltpeter, in a quart of good vinegar, and take 1 or 2 tablespoons 3 or 4 times a day.

When the gums are much swollen, with considerable ulceration, and the mouth, teeth and breath, have a fetid or bad smell, the mouth must be frequently washed with water, prepared as follows: boil red oak bark in water, then strain the water well, and in it dissolve a lump of alum, to which add a teaspoon of finely powdered charcoal.

Drink freely of an infusion made with scurvy-grass [*Cochlearia officinalis*], or eat the greens in salads, etc.

SKIN

CHAFED SKIN

Excoriation and rawness of infant skin: keep parts dry and dusted with fine powdered starch.

Wash parts well with boracic acid water. Dry thoroughly and dust with fuller's earth.

Toast wheat flour until brown; tie in rag and dust irritated parts.

Wash carefully and absorb moisture with soft dry cloth. Then apply pulverized hemlock tree bark or fuller's earth.

CHAPPED HANDS

Wash hands with Castile soap; apply it with a flannel, and, if necessary, use a brush, in order to get the dirt from under and around the nails and fingers, till they are perfectly clean; then rinse them in a little clean water, and, while they are wet, rub them well all over with about ½ tablespoon of good honey; then dry them well, with a clean coarse towel. This should be done once or twice a day, and always before going to bed. After washing clean, apply vinegar, and put on your gloves on going to bed.

Wash them with soft soap, mixed with red sand, or, wash them in sugar and water.

Instead of using soap for washing the hands, use oatmeal; and after wiping the hands, use a little dry oatmeal to rub over them, to absorb the moisture.

The seeds of quince soaked in warm water afford a soothing lotion for chapped or cracked skin.

Simmer together beeswax, balm gilead buds and sheep tallow.

To prevent chapped hands. Wash them with flour of mustard, or in bran and water boiled together.

FRECKLES

Scald some meadowsweet [*Spiraea ulmaria*] with boiling water. Allow to cool, then strain. Wash the face with this frequently.

Bruise and then squeeze the juice out of the common chickweed, and to this juice add 3 times its quantity of soft water. Bathe the skin with this for 5 to 10 minutes, and wash afterwards with clean water, night and morning. Elder flowers may be treated and applied exactly in the same manner. When the flowers are not to be had, the distilled water from them will answer the purpose.

The seeds of marshmallow, either green or dry, mixed with vinegar, will clear the skin of discolorings, by being bathed with it in the sun.

FUNGUS

An external application of the powdered bloodroot destroys fungus flesh, and heals sores of long standing.

Take soft soap and bayberry. Mix well together and form a plaster.

Apply the juice of garlic to affected parts.

Make a strong decoction of dried or fresh elder leaves and apply to affected parts.

IMPETIGO

Apply the fresh mashed leaves of impetigo bush [*Cassia alata*].
West Indies slave recipe

Apply the fresh mashed leaves or the dried powdered leaves of common plantain or the powdered roots of golden seal root.

Apply the extract of grindelia [*Grindelia robusta* or *G. squarrosa*].

PIMPLES

Oil of juniper applied, will dry them up.

Take a teaspoon of alum to a quart of water and use as a wash 3 times a day.

Take a teaspoon of the tincture of gum guaiacum, and 1 teaspoon of vinegar; mix, and apply it to the affected parts.

PRICKLY HEAT

Mix a large portion of wheat bran with either cold or lukewarm water, and use it as a bath twice or thrice a day. Children who are covered with prickly heat in warm weather will be thus effectually relieved from that tormenting eruption. As soon as it begins to appear on the neck, face and arms, commence using the bran water on these parts repeatedly through the day, and it may spread no further. If it does, the bran water bath will certainly cure it, if persisted in.

Bathe parts with baking soda and water, dry thoroughly and apply talcum.

Bathe 2 or 3 times a day with warm water, in which a moderate quantity of bran and common soda has been stirred. After wiping the skin dry, dust the affected parts with cornstarch.

Dust parts with browned cornstarch.

Bathe parts with cool salt water.

Take 1 ounce powdered borax, 2 ounces cologne, 1 quart alcohol, 3 quarts rainwater; bathe with solution 3 times a day.

A mixture of vinegar and water will often relieve the heat and burning.

Wash parts with a strong decoction of white oak bark. After drying, dust with starch or oatmeal.

A nice wash for the delicate skin of infants is made by obtaining maple twigs. Put in a small lump of alum and boil the twigs. Wash the tender places with this in lieu of water.

Adults: carry a piece of alum in pocket.

RASH

Make a decoction of celandine herb with a little sal soda and use as a wash.

A mixture of olive oil, vinegar, and spirits of wine, affords relief.

Apply fresh juice of *Aloe vera*.

Nettle rash may be cured by rubbing the part affected with fresh rosemary, mint, sage or yellow dock leaves.

Drink a tea made of cudweed and use a strong decoction of the same herb as a wash.

Take grated turnip and radish, plus finely chopped onion, and a level teaspoon each of aniseed and sulphur, mixed together and taken 3 times a day. This will go far in clearing up rashes common in spring.

SCARS

Coconut oil, or hen's oil, applied to a scar and rubbed gently for 5 minutes at a time, several times a day, will entirely obliterate a scar if commenced from the time the burn heals. The rubbing will loosen the skin and flesh from the bone and muscle and cause circulation. Even where the scar is of long standing this will be of much assistance, and perseverance will work wonders in scars left by cut, burn or bruise.

Miss M. C. Cooke, 1889

SUNBURN

Apply juice of lemon or lime, vinegar, and olive oil or vaseline, mixed with enough menthol to make a cooling salve.

Apply juice of *Aloe vera*.

Wash face with decoction made of sage leaves.

SLIVERS or SPLINTERS

For thorns, wood, steel or glass splinters, apply poultice of raw bacon.

Small splinters. Nearly fill a wide mouthed bottle with hot water, place the injured part over the mouth of the bottle and press tightly. The suction will draw the flesh down and in a minute or 2 the steam will extricate the splinter. If the above does not work press out splinter with fingers. The steam softens the skin area where splinter is.

To remove splinters or briars, place a piece of adhesive tape over the wound before retiring. By morning the splinter or briar is usually sticking to the tape.

The mashed fresh leaves of marshmallow beaten with niter and applied draws out thorns and prickles.

Take elder root and the seed of Jamestown weed and fry it in lard. It will draw any splinters out of the flesh, or anything else in man.

SORES and SURFACE ULCERS

Apply to the sore a batch of common tow [coarse hemp or flax fiber], and keep it wet with new milk.

Dr. A. A. Benezet, 1826

Make a poultice by boiling carrots until soft and mash them to a pulp, add lard or sweet oil sufficient to keep it soft.

Make a bread and milk poultice in the usual way, then sprinkle finely powdered charcoal over it and apply. Valuable for cleansing old sores and for arresting mortification.

For sores without inflammation. Take ½ pound of the oil of spike, 1 pound of mutton tallow, 1 pound of hog's lard, heat them over a moderate fire till they are melted, then add a little rosin and beeswax, which will make it to a salve. This will cure all common sores.

The bark of white pine is a great medicine for sores. It should be boiled, and the soft part stript out and beat to a poultice in a mortar, and then sufficiently moistened with the liquor and applied to burns, or sores of any kind. Repeat the poultices and wash with the liquor until the sore is well. This will not terrify or smart in its application; a new skin will come on quickly, without a scar.

P. Smith, 1812

Take 1 pound of beeswax; 1 pound of salt butter; and 2 pounds of white pine turpentine—melt them together; then strain it off for use. Fir balsam may be added. To be spread on lint, and applied to fresh wounds or old sores. It possesses both a drawing and healing quality.

Dr. D. Rogers, 1824

Fill a 4 ounce bottle ¼ full of balm of gilead buds, fill up the bottle with alcohol. Let stand a week. The result is a tincture in many respects superior to arnica for raw sores.

The green part of the stalk of common elder mixed with sweet cream is excellent for a sore where the humors prevail.

Take 1 pound lard, ½ pound rosin, 10 ounces elder bark, boil over a slow fire for ½ hour, then strain and put into small tin boxes.

Externally, the indigofera may be applied in poultice, wash, fomentation or ointment, to ulcers of every description, but particularly to those which are in a mortifying, or mortified state, being considered by some as the most powerful antiseptic or preventive of mortification known.

H. Howard, 1857

Slippery elm powder, mixed with pounded cracker and ginger makes

229

the best poultice I have ever found; for burns, scalds, felons, old sores, etc.

S. Thomson, 1831

Break an egg and put the white in a cup, add a teaspoon of brown sugar and 1½ teaspoons of powdered slippery elm bark. Stir and mix. Do not heat. Cover the sore with a thin coating of the mixture and change frequently.

Chop fresh chickweed and boil in lard. Strain and bottle for use.

Take equal parts of chickweed and wood sage, pound together and use as poultice. It may also be prepared as in the preceding recipe.

Take wormwood herb, smartweed, blue vervain; boil in weak lye; apply with a soft brush or feather.

Poultices made of powdered comfrey root are wonderful on old sores and surface ulcers.

A strong decoction of the bark of prickly ash is used with great success, as a wash for old and foul ulcers, which it always greatly cleanses, and disposes them to heal up.

The powder of bloodroot sprinkled on an old ulcer, will cleanse it effectually from scurf, canker, and fungus flesh, and produce a healthy appearance.

Dr. D. Rogers, 1824

An application of the fresh sliced roots of poke promotes the discharge of foul ulcers.

J. Monroe, 1824

Boil the leaves of walnut tree in soft water, and frequently wash the sore with it, keeping a cloth wet with the wash on the parts all the time.

Make a strong decoction of white oak bark. Use as a wash for ulcers and old sores—it cannot be surpassed.

Apply poultice made of fresh stalks of common horsetail grass, or make a wash of a strong decoction of the dried herb.

Bayberry bark of root used in the form of a poultice is a sovereign remedy in scrofulous ulceration.

Water dock roots made into a strong decoction by boiling in water, or an ointment made by simmering the root in hog's lard is a valuable remedy, derived from the Indians.

J. C. Gunn, M.D., 1830

An ointment may be made by simmering white or yellow melilot in fresh butter, or lard, which is of great use in foul ulcers and old sores.

Boil 2 ounces of the root of white pond lily to 1 pint of water for 20 minutes. Gently apply the lotion when cooled to sores or ulcers with a small piece of cotton wool, which should be used once only and burned. This is also a good lotion for many other kinds of sores and blotches.

Mashed fresh botanicals that have been used as poultices on sores: common plantain leaves, calendula flowers or leaves, self-heal herb, burdock leaves, yerba mansa, gum plant leaves, and many other non-toxic green leaves.

SPRAINS

Sprains are best treated with hot water. Pour it from a distance upon the sprained joint. Use water as hot as can be borne, persisting until the inflammation and swelling have subsided. Then bandage and use some simple remedy.

The white of an egg, and salt mixed to a thick paste is one of the best remedies for sprains, or bruises, or lameness, for man or beast. Rub well the part affected.

Take 1 ounce of ginger, the whites of 2 eggs, and 1 teaspoon of fine salt; make these into a poultice and lay it on the parts affected.

Use a tablespoon of honey, the same quantity of fine bay salt, and the white of a hen's egg. Beat the whole up together for 2 hours at least. Let it stand 1 hour and anoint the sprained part with the oil which is produced from the mixture, keeping it well bound with a flannel bandage. This will generally enable a person to walk free from pain in 1 day.

Take the whites of 3 hens' eggs, ½ pint of vinegar, 2 spoonsful of salt, beat well together and apply to the parts affected; bathe them well, and put on flannel.

Take the white of an egg and teaspoon each of vinegar and spirits of turpentine. Put into bottle, shake thoroughly, then bathe sprain often, beginning as soon as possible after the accident.

Cider vinegar, kerosene and salt, mixed, make a good house liniment for sprains and swellings, etc.

Make a poultice with vinegar and bran or with the addition of oatmeal, or bread crumbs. As poultice dries out moisten with vinegar.

Apply a poultice made of stiff clay and vinegar.

Fill a pint jar with lobelia herb; add ½ teaspoon powdered cayenne pepper and cover with pure cider vinegar. Let stand tightly closed for 3 days, shaking occasionally. Strain and use as a liniment applied to the affected parts.

Make pounded resin into a paste with fresh butter, lay it on the sprained part and bind it up.

Bruise the fresh stalks of wormwood, moisten with vinegar, and apply to sprain.

Make a liniment strong as possible with good vinegar and wormwood, adding a piece of saltpeter the size of a hickory nut to ½ pint of the liquid.

Mix 1 teaspoon oil of wormwood with 1 pint of rubbing alcohol. Apply to sprain or bruise—keep a cloth wet with it on injured part.

The green herb of wormwood pounded, and a tincture made from the same, with spirit, is excellent for bruises and sprains.

The bark of the root of bittersweet with chamomile and wormwood simmered in fresh lard makes an excellent ointment.

Take tansy, wormwood, horehound herb, catnip, and hops, of each an equal quantity. Bruise them and put them into a kettle, cover over with spirits and lard, and let it stand 2 weeks; then simmer awhile and strain. Add 1 pound of common white turpentine, to every 10 pounds of the ointment. This ointment is very cooling, resolvent, relaxing, and emollient. It is very useful in sprains, contusions, swellings, dislocations, contracted sinews, etc.

W. Beach, M.D., 1833

Oil of sassafras will cure a sprain if bathed thoroughly and bound with a thick bandage of flannel.

These are best treated with showerings of water, after which do them up in bandages wrung out in arnica and water or witch hazel and water. In all cases keep bandages moist, without undoing them. Absolute rest for the injured point is a prime necessity.

Hot fomentations of life everlasting have been used like arnica for sprains and bruises, and form a good vulnerary for painful tumors and unhealthy ulcers.

C. F. Millspaugh, M.D., 1887

Take of bittersweet bark of root, pellitory-of-the-wall, mullein flowers, 1 pound of each, all fresh, bruise them and add 1 gallon of bear's oil, or any other soft oil; simmer the whole in an earthen or iron vessel 6 hours, over a slow fire; then strain it off, add 1 pint of spirits of turpentine, and keep it close corked for use. To be applied to sprains, bruises, contracted tendons, etc.

Dr. D. Rogers, 1824

The leaves of common burdock wilted will ease pain, and pounded green and applied externally will afford relief to a bruise or sprain.

P. F. Bowker, 1836

STIFFNESS

NECK

Fill a bag with hot salt and sleep on it.

Rub neck with oil of sassafras.

JOINTS

Dissolve camphor gum in olive oil, and rub stiffened joint with this preparation, 3 or 4 times daily.

Take of the bark of white oak and bark of sweet apple trees, equal parts; boil them down to a thick substance, and then add the same quantity of goose grease or oil; simmer all together, and then rub it on the parts warm.

Dr. A. A. Benezet, 1826

Take 1 pound of hog's lard, put into it a small handful of white melilot or yellow clover, stew it well together, strain it off and add to it 1 ounce rattlesnake grease, 1 ounce olive oil, 10 drops oil of lavender, mixed well together. Anoint 3 times a day and rub parts well.

Dr. L. Sperry, 1843

STOMACH DISTRESS

ACIDITY, HEARTBURN OR SOUR STOMACH

Dissolve 1 teaspoon salt in ½ wineglass of water and drink.

Take a swallow of hickory limb ashes and water 3 times a day.

To 1 quart of hickory ashes add 6 ounces of wood soot. Put them into a gallon of boiling water, let it stand for 12 hours and then bottle for use. Take from 1 tablespoon to a wineglassful 15 minutes after each meal.

Take of quick lime, 2 ounces, and of pure water, 5½ pints: mix—let them steep 2 hours in an earthen vessel; then pour off the clear water, and keep it closely corked in bottles for use. Dose—½ a gill may be taken at once, several times a day, in an empty stomach. It corrects acidity of the stomach, and dissolves discharges and redundancy of slime and mucus, which affords a lodgement for worms. A tablespoon may be added to ½ pint of milk, to make it sit easy in weak stomachs.

Dr. D. Rogers, 1824

The best remedy is to use refined chalk, or if this cannot be had, use common chalk. Take the meat of peach stones, or peach leaves or bark from the root of black cherry tree, dried and pounded fine. Use a teaspoon of the powder and the same quantity of chalk, in a glass of hot water after eating. It will be found an excellent preventive of these disorders.

P. F. Bowker, 1836

Lobelia if properly taken, is usually an effectual cure for this disease. It should be frequently taken in honey, in as large doses as the stomach will bear, and upon an empty stomach. Oyster shells, and other medicines of the same class, in many cases might with propriety be used. Equal quantities of beef's gall and chalk, taken in doses of a teaspoon, 3 times a day, is very efficacious. The gall should be dried and powdered, and mixed with the chalk.

Dr. L. Sperry, 1843

Chew calamus or slippery elm bark and swallow the juice.

Grandmother's favorite remedy for sour stomach or heartburn was horehound candy.

F. M. G.

An infusion made with black horehound is often effective against acidity.

FLATULENCE OR GAS

Stir level teaspoon ground ginger in ½ glass of hot water for 2 or 3 minutes and strain. Add ½ teaspoon of baking soda and drink.

Take a teaspoon of activated charcoal with as little water as possible to get it down.

Pennyroyal tea is good to restore the wanted heat of the stomach. It will remove wind in the stomach, and may be used without fear, as it is perfectly harmless.

Chew saffron flowers and swallow the spittle.

CRAMPS CAUSED BY FLATULENCE OR GAS

When the cramp is located in the stomach or bowels, flannels dipped in hot water, wrung out, and laid over the parts affected, relieve the pain.

Take a teaspoon of saleratus pulverized, 1 tablespoon of molasses, stir it well together, take it all at a dose.

Friction should be immediately employed where the pain is, and continued until a degree of heat is produced, and the pain subsides. Should this fail of giving relief, administer ½ teaspoon of red pepper in ½ tumbler of water or tea; also peppermint tea, or, as a substitute, any common herb tea. Bathe the feet in warm water, and apply a heated brick, covered with a cloth and wet with vinegar, to the breast, as hot as can be borne.

Mrs. E. A. Howland, 1847

Drink an infusion made with peppermint herb and water or with peppermint steeped in hot (not boiling) milk. This may be given to children or infants in teaspoonful doses while tea or milk are warm.

The warm infusion made with either fennel seed or caraway seed is very soothing to infants. The infusion may be slightly sweetened.

Ginseng root is good for the stomach, infused in a little spirit; the dry root grated in hot water, and sweetened, is good for children in case of pain in the stomach and bowels, caused by wind. It is a safe remedy also for weakness.

Tea made from silverweed is an excellent remedy in attacks of cramp, in the stomach, abdomen, or elsewhere. When symptoms of the cramp first appear, the patient should be given 3 times daily, very warm milk (as warm as possible) in which such herbs (as much as can be taken with 3 fingers) have been boiled as for tea. A greater effect may be obtained if at the same time as the tea is taken, a poultice is made of the boiled herbs, and laid upon the afflicted part.

German recipe

Take a pint of the decoction of ground ivy with a teaspoon of the same herb powdered, 5 or 6 mornings.
The American Family Receipt Book, 1854

Swallow 5 or 6 grains of white pepper for 6 or 7 mornings.

Lady slipper root has a bracing quality, and is good.

A decoction of the roots or seeds of angelica will be useful; or ⅙ part teaspoon of cayenne, in a gill of hot water; or a tea made of the flowers of mullein.
Dr. D. Rogers, 1824

Take 1 or 2 teaspoons tincture of prickly ash berries 3 times a day.

Take the oil of lavender, and put 10 drops on loaf sugar or in a little wine. If this does not give immediate relief, repeat the dose in an hour. It very rarely fails.

Dissolve oil of cajeput, oil of cloves, oil of peppermint, oil of anise, each, 1 fluid drachm, in rectified alcohol 4 fluid ounces. This is useful in colic, cramp of the stomach, or elsewhere, flatulence, pains in the stomach or bowels, painful diarrhea, cholera morbus, Asiatic cholera, and in all cases where a stimulant and antispasmodic is required. The dose is from 20 drops to a fluid drachm, in some sweetened water in simple syrup or mucilage of slippery elm.

J. King, M.D., 1864

INDIGESTION OR DYSPEPSIA

There is nothing like hot water for this distress. The following item is from the Hartford *Courant,* which has proven in hundreds of cases to be very valuable. Use the hot water 1 hour before each meal, instead of only at breakfast. "A gentleman who is in business in this city has cured himself of a chronic and ugly form of dyspepsia in a very simple way. He was given up to die; but he finally abandoned alike the doctors and the drugs, and resorted to a method of treatment which most doctors and most persons would laugh at as an 'old woman's remedy.' It was simply swallowing 1 teacup hot water before breakfast every morning. He took the water from the cook's teakettle, and so hot that he could only take it by the spoonful. For about 3 weeks this morning dose was repeated, the dyspepsia decreasing all the while. At the end of that time he could eat, he says, any breakfast or dinner that any well person could eat—had gained in weight, and has ever since been hearty and well. His weight is now between 30 and 40 pounds greater than it was during the dyspepsia sufferings; and for several years he has had no trouble with his stomach—unless it was some temporary inconvenience due to a late supper or dining out, and in such case a single trial of his ante-breakfast remedy was sure to set all things right. He obtained his idea from a German doctor, and in turn recommended it to others—and in every case, according to this gentleman's account, a cure was effected."

Mrs. M. W. Ellsworth, 1897

Drink hot water in which a small teaspoon of salt has been dissolved.

Drink a ½ glass of water in which has been put the juice of a lemon (no sugar) morning and evening.

Drink a glass of water to which has been added ½ teaspoon bicarbonate of soda and 10 or 12 drops essence of peppermint.

Boil ½ pint of white wheat 3 hours in a quart of water, or a little more if necessary. Drink ½ pint of the liquid 2 or 3 times a week.

Mrs. E. A. Howland, 1847

Swallow the yolk of 1 egg with a little salt before breakfast.

Take chicken gizzard's peelings, dry them, pulverize them and take a teaspoon at a dose and it will answer a good purpose in a relaxed state.

Dr. L. Sperry, 1843

White mustard seed is good when swallowed whole in doses of 1 teaspoon at a time before eating.

Put a tablespoon of whole white mustard seed in 2 ounces of molasses. Take 1 or 2 tablespoons once a day.

Steep ½ ounce of hops in 1 pint of boiling water for 10 minutes. Strain. Drink a wineglassful before meals.

Take 1 pint of wild black cherries, steep in 1 pint of old Jamaica spirits. Take ½ wineglassful twice a day. Use no sugar. This has accomplished wonderful cures. Avoid all spirits after you have regained your usual health.

The bark of the root of prickly ash is a splendid tonic. Use as a tincture in whisky—generally used along with other articles such as poke root and gum guaiac. As a stimulating bitters, probably nothing better grows in the forest than prickly ash. Take of the powder, either of the bark of root or of the berries, 10 to 30 grains, about 3 times a day.

Dr. R. L. Louis, 1877

The bark of black alder made into a syrup, is good for those troubled with indigestion.

Steep 1 or 2 teaspoons of dried wormwood herb in 1 pint of boiling water for 3 or 4 minutes. Strain. Take 1 to 4 teaspoons daily.

Pour boiling water on 2 ounces of chamomile flowers, and stand till cold; strain, and add a little carbonate of soda, and take 1 tablespoonful 3 times a day.

Samphire is a very good herb and was used more in former times than it is now. It is well known to almost every one that ill digestion and obstructions are the cause of most of the diseases which the frail nature of man is subject to. Both might be remedied in a measure by a more frequent use of this herb. It is a safe herb, very pleasant, both to taste and stomach.

Steep ½ teaspoon of quassia chips in a tumbler of water. Take a swallow before meals. Refill the tumbler 2 or 3 mornings and then take new chips or take 1 ounce quassia chips, ½ pint of gin, ½ pint water. Put in a bottle and do not use until the chips settle. Take 1 tablespoon before eating.

Take dried roots of lovage, half a drachm at a time, powdered and in wine, 3 times a day before eating. It helps to warm a cold stomach, and clears it of all raw and superfluous moisture, which always exists when a person is troubled with indigestion. Want of action at the stomach is the cause. Any thing therefore which will produce an action by warming the stomach and assisting it to throw off the cold and superfluous saliva, must, according to the nature of things, be beneficial in such cases.

P. F. Bowker, 1836

Chew a small piece of gentian root and swallow the juice.

Gentian root 1 ounce; orange peel 1 ounce; fresh lemon peel 1 ounce; rhubarb root 1 grain; sal soda 1 grain. Steep in 1 quart of boiling water. Take 1 tablespoon before eating.

Take ½ ounce each of gentian, black alder, wild black cherry bark and orange peel. Steep in ½ pint of boiling water. When cool, strain and add ½ pound sugar and 1 quart sweet wine. Bottle tightly. Take a wineglassful 3 times a day.

Spearmint 2 ounces; powdered ginger 1½ ounces; columbo 1½ ounces; gentian 1 ounce; canella bark ¾ ounce; gin 1½ pints. Mix and pour upon them 1½ pints of boiling water; add as much tincture of capsicum as will make the tonic pleasantly warm. Take from 1 to 2 tablespoons before meals.

Dr. B. W. James, 1852

Take 1 ounce gentian root; Peruvian bark 1 ounce; ½ ounce orange peel, ½ ounce coriander seed. Steep in 1 quart French brandy and let it stand 4 or 5 days before using. Take from ½ teaspoon to a teaspoon in a wineglass of water about an hour before meals.

H. R. Stout, M.D., 1886

Golden seal root is useful to remove the heavy, disagreeable sensation often produced by indigestible food. Take a teaspoon of powdered root in hot water—sweeten.

Take of golden seal a teaspoon, poplar bark 2 teaspoons, sugar 4 teaspoons, red pepper ⅛ teaspoon. Have all these in powder; mix them together, and about ½ hour, or an hour, after dinner, take ½ teaspoon of the mixture in some water, repeating it in ½ hour or 1 hour, if necessary.

Take of golden seal, black alder bark, Solomon's seal, in coarse powder, a tablespoon; boiling water 1 pint; mix, and steep near a hot fire for 6 hours; strain, and sweeten to suit the taste. Of this, a tablespoon may be taken every 2 or 3 hours, in the beginning of the attack.

Take of golden seal root; tulip tree bark, bitter-root, each, bruised, 1 drachm; prickly ash berries, sassafras bark, capsicum, each ½ drachm; sherry wine 3 pints. Macerate for 14 days, with occasional agitation; then express and filter. Dose from ½ to 2 fluid ounces, 3 times a day.

J. King, M.D., 1864

Take 1 dram pulverized golden seal root; 2 drams white wood bark; Indian hemp; ½ dram cayenne pepper or capsicum and 1 quart sweet Malaga wine. Add all to wine and allow to infuse for a few days. Take from ¼ to ½ wineglass 3 or 4 times a day.

W. Beach, M.D., 1833

Follow a strict diet. Drink an infusion made with the following mixture: ½ ounce each of meadowsweet herb, balmony herb, barberry bark, centaury herb, calamus root, ½ ounce wormwood herb. Add 1 teaspoon powdered capsicum or ginger to mixture.

Take 1 ounce powdered rhubarb root, 1 ounce caraway seed, 1 tablespoon grated orange peel. Put into a decanter with 1 pint of best brandy, shake it well together, and keep in a warm place. Take 1 tablespoon in the morning, fasting, and at night going to bed. Shake the mixture well before taking it.

J. Marquart, 1867

Boil 1 ounce mayapple root in 1 pint of water for 5 minutes. Take 1 tablespoon 5 or 6 times daily if possible [as mayapple is cathartic, it probably is only useful when dyspepsia is caused by constipation.]

Mayapple root, blue flag root and dogbane 1 ounce each in very fine powder, blood root, fine, ½ ounce, red pepper fine, 2 drams, saleratus 1 ounce; dose, ½ teaspoon in water 3 times a day.

C. Kinsley, 1876

NERVOUS, UPSET OR STRAINED STOMACH

Boil ½ cup barley in plain water slowly and set aside to cool. Make this liquid produce 3 cups. Drink warm on empty stomach.

Take ⅛ pound of pitch from the end of a white pine log, the same quantity of sulphur, and ½ pound of honey; simmer well together, take 2 pills of this every day before eating. There is but one chance in this medicine for a person to be disappointed. That is, it generally effects a cure before the medicine is ½ used up.

P. F. Bowker, 1836

Drink a decoction made with water and the bark of peach tree.

Chamomile tea has proved most useful for dyspepsia brought on by fit of passion, anger especially of sensitive females. The warm tea is also useful for cramps.

WEAK OR SICK STOMACH

Hot water is excellent in cases of sick stomach, and may be taken when no nourishment of any kind can be retained in the stomach.

For a person that has been troubled with a weak stomach for a long time. In the first place, omit taking all kinds of medicine whatever. Take rye, wash it clean, and boil it in the same manner as you would rice. Make this your constant diet. This may be eaten with molasses, or in milk. Be sure and not take any other kind of food whatever, till you are thoroughly satisfied you can bear it. Drink a tea of white pine bark and slippery elm. This has been known to cure persons who have been troubled with a weak stomach for years, and become so much reduced as not to be able to bear ½ a cracker at a meal.

P. F. Bowker, 1836

Let your diet be milk, with a tablespoon of the best brandy you can get in it, and any kind of light bread, and drink a tea made of strawberry leaves, with a red pepper broken in it. This is a safe remedy.

Salts of tartar 30 grains, oil of mint 6 drops; powdered gum arabic, ⅛ ounce; powdered loaf sugar, ⅛ ounce; water, 6 ounces. A tablespoon of this mixture is a dose.

Boil 1 ounce of spearmint herb in a pint of water for 2 minutes. Take a tablespoon 3 or 4 times a day or whenever the sickness is felt.

Gruel made of powdered slippery elm is good for weak stomach. Gruel is made by adding slippery elm to cold water, then stir into boiling, till the thickness of gruel.

Drink frequently a tea made of boiling water and red clover flowers.

The flowers of hollyhock is very strengthening, and good for a weak stomach. They are also good in weakly female complaints, if used as a constant drink, and taken in season.

A tea made of the herb blessed thistle, taken cold, is good in a weak debilitated state of the stomach.

Chewing a piece of ginseng root and swallowing the juice is a pleasant tonic for weakness of the stomach and indigestion.

Drink 3 or 4 times a day, of the steep made from the bark of white poplar roots.

Eat cooked or raw the inner bark or root of birch.

A teaspoon of the powdered root of American colombo in hot water and sugar will give immediate relief in case of heavy food loading a weak stomach.

C. S. Rafinesque, 1828

Chamomile flowers when steeped in old whiskey, or any good spirits, and taken 2 or 3 times a day, in moderate quantities, is an excellent medicine to give tone or strength to a weak stomach and restore the appetite.

J. C. Gunn, M.D., 1830

Wild ginger root steeped in very little spirit is good.

Take 1 ounce of calumbo root, add an 1½ ounce horehound, 1 ounce poplar bark, and 1 ounce of red raspberry leaves; boil the whole in 1 quart of water and when strained add ½ teaspoon of cayenne pepper. Dose, ½ wineglassful 3 or 4 times a day.

Take of gum mastic and spermaceti, each 2 ounces; melt them together over a slow fire; then stir in brown sugar, say 2 pounds; make into small balls, the size of a walnut, and take 3 per day on an empty stomach.

Take wormwood, tansy, balm of gilead bud, buds of pitch pine, each ½ ounce; steep in 1 quart of spirits. Take from a tablespoon to ½ wineglass, morning and evening.

INFLAMED STOMACH,
TO TEMPORARILY ALLAY IRRITATION

Drink an infusion made with slippery elm bark. Tea may be made with mixture of equal parts of slippery elm and arrowroot. If the powders of the botanicals are available they may be taken in milk freely.

Dissolve 4 ounces of gum arabic in 3 gills of boiling water; sweeten to suit the taste, and flavor as may be desired, with some essence.

PALLIATIVES FOR GASTRIC ULCER

Drink freely of powdered slippery elm bark mixed in either milk or water.

Powdered slippery elm taken in teaspoon doses in milk; and with fluid extract hydrastis. The hydrastis is given in 3 to 5 drop doses in a little milk, before meals 3 times daily.

Drink freely of an infusion made with cheese plant.

Drink a cupful, as needed of infusion made with okra pods, Irish moss or licorice root.

SWELLINGS in EARLY STAGES

Also see POULTICES.

Take linseed oil, 1 pound, sweet oil or fresh butter, ½ pound, put on the fire and boil, then slack the heat, and add to it 2 pounds of beeswax, 1 pound of rosin, and stir them together till cold.

WHITE OR HARD SWELLINGS

Take of rum ½ pint, warm it, then add ½ ounce of tincture of camphor, ½ ounce of laudanum, and put them into a bottle; and by frequently rubbing the parts affected with this mixture, hot as can be borne, it will soon reduce the worst kind of swellings.

Take white rose petals, elder flowers, leaves of foxglove, and of St. John's wort, a handful of each; mix them with hog's lard, and make an ointment.

Hold parts affected morning and evening, in the steam of vinegar poured on red hot coals.

SOFT, FLABBY SWELLINGS

Pump cold water on them daily or use constant frictions, or proper bandages.

SWOLLEN LIMBS

Take beech leaves 1 pailful, boil them in 4 quarts of water down to 1. Bandage the limb with flannel, keep it wet 24 hours, and it will take the inflammation out and take the swelling down.

An Indian cure for the same. Take smartweed, boil it strong, and use it as above recipe.

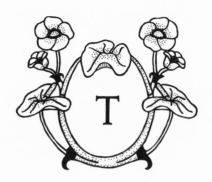

TEETH

CLEANING AND PREVENTING DECAY

Take of good soft water 1 quart; juice of lemon, 2 ounces; burnt alum, 6 grains; common salt, 6 grains. Mix. Boil them a minute, strain and bottle for use.

Mrs. E. A. Howland, 1847

Put a piece of quicklime, as big as a walnut, in a pint of water in a bottle. Clean the teeth with a little of it every morning, rinsing the mouth with clean water afterward. If the teeth are good, it will preserve them, and keep away the toothache; if the teeth are gone, it will harden the gums, so that they will masticate crusts and all.

To 4 ounces of fresh prepared lime-water add a drachm of Peruvian bark; wash the teeth with this water before breakfast and after supper; it will effectually destroy the tartar, and remove the offensive smell from those which are decayed.

There is nothing better than the Peruvian bark, used as a powder. The teeth and gums should be rubbed with this substance every morning. It hardens both the gums and the teeth, and keeps them from all impurity. All gritty substances should be avoided, lest the enamel of the teeth be worn off. The powdered charcoal makes a very good dentifrice.

G. Capron, M.D., and D. B. Slack, M.D., 1848

The wood itself, of the dogwood tree is considerably used by dentists—by which I mean tooth cleaners and setters—in putting in artificial teeth. The young branches, stripped of their bark, and rubbed with their ends against the teeth, render them extremely white and beautiful. These are tooth brushes of nature's presenting, and are infinitely better than those made of hog's bristles, and filled with snuff, and such other delightful aromatics! The negroes of the Southern States, and those of the West India Islands, who are remarkable for the whiteness of their teeth, are in the constant practice of rubbing them with the small branches of the dogwood, or of some other tree which will answer the purpose. [Small branches are pounded at the ends in order to loosen fiber and form natural brush.]

J. C. Gunn, M.D., 1830

Take the barks of bayberry, yellow oak, and black alder, equal quantities—pulverize and mix—to which may be added 1 part ginger. To be applied in the powder or decoction, with a brush or the end of the finger. It cleanses the teeth and gums from scurvy or scorbutic matter, gives the enamel a smooth polish, and a white appearance, strengthens the gums and loose teeth, and if regularly used, prevents them from decaying.

Dr. D. Rogers, 1824

It is said that the root of wintergreen chewed 6 weeks every spring by young people, totally prevents toothache.

J. Monroe, 1824

TOOTHACHE

Take of creosote or the oil of smoke, wet lint or cotton wool with this, and put it into the hollow of the tooth; and it will cure.

The worst toothache, or neuralgia coming from the teeth, may be speedily ended by the application of a small bit of clean cotton saturated in a strong solution of ammonia to the defective tooth. Sometimes the application causes nervous laughter, but the pain has disappeared.

*The Modern Home Cook Book
and Family Physician,* about 1880

Equal quantities powdered alum and fine salt applied to the tooth will give speedy relief. For an ulcerating tooth, take a piece of old, thin muslin, about 1½ inches wide and as long as desired, wet some ground flaxseed in cold water, place in the cloth, and fold and baste it together; place this upon the outside of the gum; it will soothe the pain in a short time and draw the ulcer to that spot, where it can easily be lanced.

Mrs. M. W. Ellsworth, 1897

Apply powdered alum or fill the mouth with warm water, and immediately after with cold. For inflamed face caused by toothache, apply a poultice of pounded slippery elm bark and cold water.

Practical Housekeeping, 1887

Split an onion, roast it and bind it while hot on the wrist, over the pulse, on the opposite side from the aching tooth.

One ounce alcohol, 2 drachms cayenne pepper, 1 ounce kerosene oil; mix, and let stand 24 hours—a sure cure.

Cajeput oil dropped on lint, and placed in the hollow of the tooth, or even around the gum, is generally efficacious in immediately affording ease to the sufferer. Oils of nutmeg, cinnamon, cloves or marjoram are also effective palliatives.

Steep a piece of coarse brown paper in cold vinegar, then grate ginger on it, and apply to the side of the face affected; the application to be made at bedtime, and kept on during the whole of the night.

Make a poultice of a slice of toast, saturate in alcohol and sprinkle with pepper. Apply externally.

Apply shavings of galangal spice around aching tooth.

A few drops of the tincture of benzoin on cotton, pressed into the decayed tooth will soon relieve the pain.

Chew tooth-ache-tree bark or apply mashed bark around aching tooth.

Chew the fresh leaves of common yarrow or the root of bull nettle.

If the tooth be hollow, clear it, take a piece of fresh dug bloodroot, break it open, and apply the bleeding part of the root to the marrow of the tooth. It will give immediate relief, and is an easy medicine.

Make an extract [or strong decoction] from white poplar bark; mix with it a little rum; put into your tooth, and you will soon find relief; or, take the bark of white poplar roots, boil it down to the thickness of tar; take a teaspoon of this extract, put into a glass of spirit, shake it well, and apply to the tooth.

The fibrous strings in leave stems of plantain have been extolled as an almost certain cure for aching carious teeth, if placed in the ear on the affected side. It is said these fibers turn black if the pain is relieved but remain green if not.

C. F. Millspaugh, M.D., 1887

BLEEDING FROM EXTRACTION

For bleeding at the cavity of an extracted tooth, pack the alveolus fully and firmly with cotton wet with alum water.

Make a strong decoction of horsetail grass and hold in the mouth as long as possible. Repeat with fresh decoction until bleeding stops.

TEETHING INFANTS

Great care is required in feeding young children during the time of teething. They often cry as if disgusted with food, when it is chiefly owing to the pain occasioned by the edge of a silver or metal spoon pressing on their tender gums. The spoon ought to be of ivory, bone, or wood with the edges round and smooth, and care should be taken to keep it sweet and clean. At this period a moderate looseness, and a copious flow of saliva, are favorable symptoms. With a view to promote the latter, the child should be made to gnaw such substances as tend to mollify the gums, and by their pressure to facilitate the appearance of the teeth. A piece of licorice or marshmallow root will be serviceable, or the gums may be softened and relaxed by rubbing them with honey or sweet oil.

The pain of teething may be almost done away, and the health of the child benefited by giving it very small pieces of ice, to melt in its mouth. The instant quiet which succeeds hours of fretfulness is the best witness to this magic remedy.

Make a necklace of the bean called Job's tears, and let the child wear it around the neck.

Steep 1 teaspoon of columbo in 1 cup of boiling water for 5 minutes. Strain when cold. Give to child in teaspoonful dose as needed to stop vomiting caused by teething.

Steep 1 teaspoon burdock seeds or chamomile flowers in 1 cup of boiling water. Strain after 2 or 3 minutes. Sweeten. Give to infant while still warm in teaspoon doses. For calming teething infants.

CLEANING INFANTS' TEETH

Clean them every day with borax. If a brush is too severe, try a soft cloth dipped in borax either dissolved in warm water, or pulverized: if the gums are tender it will heal and harden.

Miss T. S. Shute, 1878

THROAT

SIMPLE SORE THROAT

Gargle with water as hot as can be borne, gives great relief, even in severe cases.

Gargle with whiskey diluted with a little water and swallow a little slowly.

Gargles for sore throat are made of borax, or soda, or salt, or alum, or peroxide of hydrogen—any of these mixed with water. A few drops tincture of myrrh or listerine may be added to the borax or soda solutions. Use gargle every hour faithfully until cured.

Simply wet the finger in camphor and apply it to the tonsils every few minutes. It will relieve very quickly.

A piece of camphor gum as large as a pea, kept in the mouth until dissolved, will give relief and ofttimes cure.

Put a heaping teaspoon of sulphur into 3 tablespoons water, stir and gargle once an hour.

Mix a wineglassful of good calcined magnesia and honey, to the consistence of paste or jelly, and take a spoonful once an hour through the day for a day or two. It is cooling, healing, and a very gentle cathartic.

An excellent remedy for sore throat is brewers' yeast and honey— 4 tablespoons of the first and 1 teaspoon of the latter. Mix in a cup of water, and gargle the throat 2 or 3 times an hour.

Soak in water a small piece of bread and mix with it a pinch of cayenne pepper; roll it up in the form of a pill and swallow it. Usually in 3 hours the patient will be relieved. In aggravated cases a second dose may be requisite.

Squeeze the juice of ½ lemon, in a pint bowl, add 2 tablespoons loaf sugar, 1 teaspoon glycerine, and 1 tablespoon whiskey; pour over this boiling hot water to nearly fill the bowl, and drink hot just before going to bed.

In slight affections of the throat, where the soreness, swelling, and difficulty of swallowing are not great, and the inflammatory fever is not high, it is only necessary to confine the person to a warm dry room; to produce a gentle sweat by hot herb teas; to drink flaxseed, mullein, or slippery elm bark tea; and to gargle or wash the throat with a solution of white vitriol of the strength of eye-water.

A strong decoction of cinchona bark. It is a local remedy for malignant sore throat.

Make an infusion of selfheal herb, as if making tea, using 1 pint of water to 1 ounce of the herb. Dose: Drink very slowly a wineglassful twice or 3 times a day.

Gipsy recipe

The following, using 1 or more together, may be made into a decoction for gargling: witch hazel, alum root, beth root, eyebright, or primula.

For a swollen throat a decoction of blue violet leaves [*Viola cucullata*] and water is a tested gargle; at the same time the throat bandage may be applied in the decoction instead of pure water.

The tops and flower buds of privet made into a strong decoction with water, adding a little honey and wine after straining off the botanical, makes an excellent wash for the mouth and throat when sore and inflamed, and when the gums are apt to bleed.

Mrs. A. Matteson, 1894

When throat is sore deep down chew bark of slippery elm and swallow the juice.

Chewing cubeb berries sometimes relieves sore throat.

The sanicle root is a good remedy for sore throat. Indians use it in tea, or chew the root and swallow the juice.

Take 1 part golden seal root, ½ quantity of sumach berries. Make a strong decoction; to which add a small quantity of pulverized alum. Gargle frequently.

W. Beach, M.D., 1833

Pour 1 pint of boiling water on sumach berries, golden seal root, ½ handful of each, a teaspoon of red pepper, and 2 tablespoons salt; gargle several times a day.

J. King, M.D., 1864

In mild cases, a strong tea of the witch hazel leaves, and golden seal, with the ¼ of a teaspoon of cayenne in each dose, occasionally repeated, will generally remove it. In worse cases the throat should be gargled with the same article; at the same time keeping the neck warm by the application of a flannel cloth, or woolen cravat.

H. Howard, 1857

To 1 pint of strong sage tea add 1 tablespoon of honey and 2 table-spoons of vinegar. Use as gargle for children.

Mix 1 gill of strong apple vinegar, 1 tablespoon of common salt, 1 tablespoon of honey and ½ pod of red pepper together, boil them to a proper consistency, then pour it into ½ pint of strong sage tea, take a teaspoon occasionally and it will be found an infallible cure.

Dr. A. A. Benezet, 1826

Make a strong decoction of equal parts of sage and hyssop; to every pint add ½ ounce borax. Gargle frequently.

A similar recipe advises a little alum instead of borax and sweetening the mixture with honey.

Take equal parts of sage, peppermint, wild marjoram and selfheal. Steep 1 tablespoon of mixture to 1 cup of boiling water. Strain when cool. Gargle frequently with this liquid.

When throat is too sore to gargle, inhale steam from the following mixture: Equal parts of sage, boneset herb, catnip herb, hops, and horehound herb.

TONSILLITIS OR QUINSY

Pineapple juice taken every ½ hour will cure tonsillitis. An addition of a level teaspoon of cream of tartar is more effective.

Black currant jelly is often useful for soothing quinsy.

The oil of the rattlesnake is a sovereign remedy for quinsy taken internally. If this cannot be had, let the juice of common thistle [*Cirsium arvense*] be given, which will often cure, when other remedies fail.

J. Monroe, 1824

The placing of a small quantity of cayenne pepper, in powder, on the back part of the tongue, as near as may be to the part affected, the patient endeavoring so to breathe as not to take any of the pepper into his lungs, has produced the most decided and happy effects. The operation should be repeated at suitable intervals, until the inflammation is removed.

Simmer hops in vinegar until their strength is extracted. Strain the liquid, sweeten it with sugar, and give it frequently to the patient until relieved. This is an almost infallible remedy.

J. Marquart, 1867

Simmer a quantity of sage in a little hog's lard, and give the patient from a teaspoon to tablespoon, 3 or 4 times a day, as warm as can be borne. This is also good to apply externally, mixed with a roasted onion poultice.

Make a strong decoction with thyme herb and gargle frequently.

Boil 1 ounce cudweed in 1 pint of water for 1 minute. Dose: 1 tablespoon twice daily. May also be used to gargle.

Gipsy recipe

Indians chewed the leaves and flowers of life everlasting for quinsy.
D. F. Millspaugh, M.D., 1887

To expedite recovery, a bloodroot, myrrh and capsicum swab is helpful.

Take dried mullein leaves, break and crumble them up and put them in a pipe and smoke. Get the smoke down into the throat. Do this 2 or 3 times a day.

Inhale the fumes made with 1 tablespoon of tincture of benzoin added to 1 quart boiling water.

EXTERNAL APPLICATIONS

Cut slices of salt pork or fat bacon; simmer a few minutes in hot vinegar, and apply to throat as hot as possible. When this is taken off, as the throat is relieved, put around a bandage of soft flannel.

A slice of salt pork, covered over quite thick with red pepper, and bound on the throat on going to bed.

Take a raw onion and some salt pork, chop together, make a poultice on which put a little turpentine and wrap around the throat. Change as necessary.

Boil a small bag of white beans till they are quite soft, and bind them on the neck as hot as you can bear them, and keep them warm with hot flannels, changed often. Drink a strong tea of penny-royal, as warm as you can bear it. This will generally sweat it away in the course of 6 or 8 hours. After this, be a little careful about taking cold.

P. F. Bowker, 1836

Much benefit has been derived in some cases by the application of a poultice made by roasting fresh pokeroot in the ashes until it is softened, when it should be mashed and applied warm, several times every day.

Apply to throat hot cloths that have been wrung out in a decoction made of smartweed.

Use a light flaxseed poultice, into which has been mixed some herbal oil, such as cajuput, camphor, cloves, eucalyptus, rosemary or other oils.

Take a glass of olive or sweet oil, and ½ glass of spirits of turpentine; mix them together, and rub the throat externally, wearing flannel round it at the same time. It proves effectual when applied early.

Apply peppermint oil on the outside of the throat from well up behind the ear nearly to the chin, also just in front of the ear. Apply hot cloths if relief does not follow.

Rub throat well with mixture of oil of anise and turpentine.

HOARSENESS

Use white of an egg, thoroughly beaten, mix with lemon juice and sugar. Take teaspoon occasionally.

Gargle with white of an egg beaten to a froth in ½ glass of warmed, sweetened water.

Take the whites of 2 eggs and beat them in with 2 spoonfuls of white sugar; grate in a little nutmeg, and then add a pint of lukewarm water. Stir well and drink often.

Wrap up a piece of butter as big as a walnut in sugar, and swallow it.

Take a small quantity of dry, powdered borax, place it on the tongue, let it slowly dissolve and run down the throat.

Boil a large handful of wheat bran in a quart of water; strain, sweeten with honey, and sup of it frequently.

Take the juice of 1 lemon, with sufficient sugar to saturate, and take 1 teaspoon several times a day.

Take an ounce of gum arabic, put it into a pint of cold water, set it on the fire to dissolve, and let it simmer about 10 minutes; add to it as much loaf sugar as you like, and ½ a lemon. If the cold is acute, drink as you please; but take every 10 or 15 minutes, 2 teaspoonfuls or more, as required. This is particularly good when much coughing causes hoarseness.

Spikenard root, sliced and bruised and then steeped in a teapot containing equal parts of water and spirits, and the vapor inhaled, when sufficiently cooled, will relieve the soreness and hoarseness of the throat or lungs, when arising from a cough or cold.

Put 1 ounce horehound herb in 1 pint boiling water. Steep for 2 hours, then strain. Take wineglassful as needed.

A decoction made by boiling wild plum bark in water, strained and thickened with honey, is the best thing for hoarseness.

Mrs. E. T., 1954

Take 3 parts of green comfrey roots, 1 part of wild turnip, and 1 part skunk cabbage. Grate all into some honey, or molasses, and take a teaspoon 3 or 4 times a day.

Take nettle roots, dry them in an oven, pulverize, and mix them with an equal quantity of molasses. Take a teaspoon 2 or 3 times a day.

Boil 1 ounce black currant leaves in 1 pint of water. Strain and bottle. Take 1 tablespoon 2 or 3 times a day.

Mix scraped horseradish root with loaf sugar. After standing 24 hours, add water, boil to syrup, and strain. One teaspoon every 2 hours.

A mixture of scraped horseradish with a small portion of wheaten flour, use of this a small quantity several times a day.

Make a strong tea of horseradish and yellow dock roots, sweeten with honey, and drink freely.

Take of horseradish root, boneset leaves, each, an ounce; hot water 1 pint; mix. Steep near a fire in a covered vessel for 2 hours, add ½ pint, each, of vinegar and molasses, and simmer for 15 minutes. Dose, a tablespoonful every 1, 2, or 3 hours.

THROAT TICKLE

Swallow a few small pieces of bread crumbs.

Chew some slippery elm or ginseng root and swallow the juice.

Chew a couple of whole cloves.

Gargle with infusion made of Irish moss or chew the dried seaweed and swallow the juice.

TONICS and BITTERS

Fill a water glass ⅔ full with red wine; add 1 tablespoon of garlic, grated or chopped fine. Take a teaspoon of the mixture 4 or 5 times a day, stirring the mixture on each occasion so as to get some of the garlic and some of the liquid.

Letter, 1934

Pour 1 pint of boiling water over ½ ounce wormwood herb and let it stand until cool, then strain. Take ½ wineglass 3 times a day. Fennel seed may be added to the infusion if desired.

An infusion made of blessed thistle is an excellent bitter. It may also be taken pulverized in a little molasses.

Gold thread root is a pleasant tonic, and promotes appetite and digestion.

Golden seal root is bracing and stimulating—it restores and strengthens the appetite.

Yellow root is a strong and pleasant bitter that sits easily on the stomach.

My grandmother was a sturdy lady—her pet tea was tansy in very weak infusion.

F. M. G.

A tea made of wild black cherry pounded with the stones and steeped in hot water, sweetened with loaf sugar, to which add a little brandy, is good to restore the digestive powers and create an appetite.

Make an infusion with gentian with a little ginger. Take before meals.

Mix 4 ounces of gentian root with 2 ounces of sliced bitter oranges. Pour a quart of good brandy over mixture and bottle. The bottles should be shaken repeatedly for 3 or 4 days. Take wineglassful morning and evening.

H. F. Brown, 1914

Take 2 ounces gentian root, 1 ounce orange peel, ½ ounce Virginia snakeroot. Infuse for 3 or 4 days in 2 pints French brandy. Take a small glassful twice a day.

Take ¼ ounce gentian root, ¼ ounce chamomile flowers, ¼ ounce colombo root, ¼ ounce dried orange peel, 50 cloves bruised. Put ingredients into a jug and pour over a quart of cold water. Allow to stand 24 hours and strain. Take 3 tablespoons for a dose, fasting every morning.

Take ½ each of gentian root, butternut leaves, chamomile flowers, wormwood herb. Steep in 1 quart boiling water. Strain when cool. Take wineglass once a day. May be diluted with water or wine and taken in small doses.

Take equal parts of Rocky Mountain grape root, butternut bark, and marshmallow root and mix well. Use heaping teaspoon to each cupful of water. Boil for 15 minutes. Strain when cool. Drink 2 or 3 cupfuls a day in small doses.

Take ½ ounce each of butternut leaves, dandelion root, buckbean herb, golden seal root. Boil in 2 quarts of water for 20 minutes. Dose ½ cupful 2 or 3 times a day after meals.

Take the bitter herb [*Chelone glabra*], barberry [*Berberis vulgaris*], bark of root and poplar [*Populus tremuloides*] inner bark, equal parts, pulverized, 1 ounce of the powder to a pint of hot water and ½ a pint of spirit. For a dose take ½ wineglassful. For hot bitters add a teaspoon cayenne or ginger. This is calculated to correct the bile and create an appetite by restoring digestive powers; and may be freely used both as a restorative and to prevent disease.

Another: Take poplar [*Populus tremuloides*] bark and bark of the root of bayberry [*Myrica cerifera*], 1 pound each, and boil them in 2 gallons of water, strain off and add 7 pounds of good sugar; then scald and skim it, and add ½ pound of peachmeats [kernels of peach stones] or the same quantity of cherrystone meats, pounded fine. When cool add a gallon of good brandy; and keep it in bottles for use. Take ½ wineglassful 2 or 3 times a day. This sirup is very good to strengthen the stomach and bowels, and to restore weak patients; and is particularly useful in the dysentery, which leaves the stomach and bowels in a sore state.

S. Thomson, 1831

Take 1 handful of boneset and the same of bark of the root of bittersweet and 1 large handful of the carpenter square root. Boil in 1 gallon of water until the substance is out; then strain and add 2 tablespoons of aloes, 2 of powdered rhubarb, then add 1 pint of good alcohol or other good liquor to keep it from souring. You can add to the alcohol before putting in the bitters any kind of flavor you wish, oil of wintergreen, cinnamon or peppermint, enough to flavor the whole gallon. Good for liver complaint, general debility and dyspepsia. The dose can be increased or decreased according to how it works.

Take 1 ounce of cloves, of cinnamon 1 ounce, bitter root, of the inner bark of hemlock tree 1 ounce, well pulverized together. Add this to 2 quarts of Holland gin. For a dose, commence with a tablespoon, and increase to ½ wineglass, every morning, on an empty stomach.

SPRING TONICS

Eat all the dandelion greens you can or eat all the fresh wild leeks tops you can.

The buds of the sweet apple tree, infused in rum or cider, are excellent for correcting the humors, and sweetening the blood and juices, especially in the spring of the year.

An old-fashioned and reliable spring purifying tonic is made by mixing together, ½ and ½, powdered sulphur and syrup or molasses. Dose: 1 teaspoon every morning before breakfast for 1 week. When taking this tonic guard against catching cold as this treatment will open the pores of the skin.

Sassafras tea, drunk freely in the spring, is a great blood purifier. It may be drunk hot or cold, and sweetened to taste. Some prefer a slice of lemon added to it. It is a very refreshing and palatable drink.

Black alder bark as a decoction, is an excellent drink the beginning of spring, because of its purifying and exhilarating qualities. It ought to be esteemed as a jewel.

A decoction made with Oregon grape roots (½ ounce of root boiled in 1 quart of water for 10 minutes). Taken 3 times a day in wineglassful doses it is said to be a far superior blood purifier and spring tonic.

Avens is good in the spring, to open obstructions of the liver. The juice of the fresh root or the powder of the dried root, has the same effect as the decoction. It is very safe; you need not have the dose prescribed. It is very fit to be kept in everyone's house.

Take 6 or 8 common elder leaves, cut them up small and make a tea with a pint of water. Boil 10 minutes. Take daily 1 cup fasting an hour before breakfast. Elder flowers also purify, and it would be good if in every home dispensary a box of the dried flowers were kept.

Mix together ½ ounce each of dandelion root, gentian root, prickly ash bark, red clover flowers, hops, and Jacob's ladder. This will make 1 quart. Steep in 1½ quarts boiling water for 3 minutes, then strain, and when cold add 1 pint molasses. Keep in a cool place. Take ½ wineglass 3 times a day.

Take 1 ounce each of dandelion root, yellow dock root, prickly ash bark, wintergreen leaves, gentian root, boldo leaves, Jacob's ladder, and cascara bark. Put all together in a porcelain container in 2 quarts of water and let it simmer slowly on top of the stove for about 2 hours, then strain and add sugar or molasses to suit taste. Take a wineglass 2 or 3 times a day. Half of this quantity may be made at a time. Care must be taken to keep mixture in a cool place.

A. M. S. family

Purchase from the druggist about 5¢ worth each of sassafras, sarsaparilla, yellow dock, burdock root, and dandelion root. Mix well together and put about 1 generous handful of this mixture into 1 quart water and boil 2 hours. Dose, 1 small wineglassful 3 times a day.

Take 1 ounce mayapple root, 1 ounce dandelion roots, 1 ounce burdock roots, 1 ounce yellow dock roots, 2 ounces prickly ash berries, 1 ounce marshmallow roots, ½ ounce rhubarb, 1 ounce gentian, 1 ounce chamomile, 2 ounces red clover flowers. Put all in an earthen crock and pour over 2 quarts of water that has been boiled and allowed to cool. Let stand overnight. Next morning place under low fire, for ½ hour. Strain and add 1 pint of gin. Take 1 teaspoon before meals.

Mrs. H. C., 1956

Recommended for sallow complexion acquired through the long, dark winter days. Take ½ ounce each of spruce, hemlock, sarsaparilla root, dandelion root, burdock root, and yellow dock root. Boil in 1 gallon of water for ½ an hour, strain while hot and add 10 drops each of oil of spruce and oil of sassafras, mix thoroughly. When cold, add ½ pound brown sugar, and ½ cup yeast. Let stand 12 hours in a jar covered tight—then bottle. Use freely as an iced drink.

Practical Housekeeping, 1887

SPRING TONICS FOR LADIES AND CHILDREN

Take 1 ounce red clover flowers, 1 ounce raspberry leaves, ½ ounce agrimony herb and enough cinnamon to flavor. Prepare the mixture like Chinese tea.

An infusion made with the herb speedwell is one of the best medicines for children in the spring.

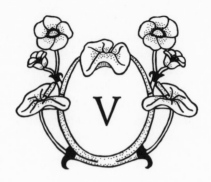

VOMITING

Ice dissolved in the mouth often cures vomiting when all remedies fail. Much depends on the diet of persons liable to such attacks; this should be easily digestible food, taken often and in small quantities. Vomiting can often be arrested by applying a mustard paste over the region of the stomach. It is not necessary to allow it to remain until the parts are blistered, but it may be removed when the part becomes thoroughly red, and reapplied if required after the redness has disappeared. One of the secrets to relieve vomiting is to give the stomach perfect rest, not allowing the patient even a glass of water, as long as the tendency remains to throw it up again.

Mix salt and vinegar together, give a teaspoon every few minutes.

For nausea threatening vomiting, take from a teaspoon to a tablespoon of lime-water with equal amount of milk, water, or cinnamon water.

Take field corn and parch it as brown as you can get it without burning. When parched put it in boiling water and drink the water as often as necessary.

Take clean cobs, burn them until they are red, then put them into water, let them soak until the strength is out, then drink of the liquor, and it will cure; it is good for summer complaint.

Dr. L. Sperry, 1843

An infusion of oatmeal made into a cake with water, then burned like coffee, will check vomiting.

An old recipe used by a doctor on a very sick patient: peel a large onion and cut in half. Place ½ in each armpit. According to this source: In several attacks since that time have I seen this remedy promptly control the incessant vomiting, and relieve the distressing nausea.

C. H. Fowler and W. H. DePuy, 1880

A syrup made of quinces with sugar is excellent to stop vomiting and to strengthen the stomach.

An infusion made of ginger, allspice, cinnamon or cloves will often stop vomiting.

A tea made either of the green or dried leaves of horsemint will stop vomiting, or puking—especially in bilious fevers. Steep 1 teaspoon of leaves in cup of boiling water for 4 or 5 minutes. Drink a wineglassful at a time.

J. C. Gunn, M.D., 1830

Bruise fresh peppermint leaves and apply to the stomach.

Chew the fresh leaves of spearmint or drink a tea made of the dried leaves. Sweeten if desired.

Take of the bruised spearmint herb a sufficient quantity, or the essence of spearmint, add to brandy and loaf sugar enough to make palatable. Very good to check vomiting.

People weakened by illness, seized with palpitation at every trifle, suffering much from nausea and frequent vomiting, should frequently make use of mint tea and mint powder.

Make an infusion of chamomile and add a little mint to the tea. Sweeten and sip.

Chamomile tea is excellent for weak stomach, to stop vomiting.

Take green wheat or green grass, pound it and pour on boiling water, and sweeten with loaf sugar. Press out the juice, and let the patient drink a tablespoon every 10 minutes.

A drink made of common pigweed is said to be a good remedy. The leaves of the plant were used by Indians for stomach ailments.

Pour boiling water on a piece of camphor, and take 1 dessertspoonful every 10 minutes, until the vomiting ceases.

Take a teaspoon of powdered columbo root every 3 or 4 hours: or as a decoction, or tea, a wineglassful 3 or 4 times a day: or steep 2 ounces of the root in a quart of old whiskey, which must stand for a few days, that the spirits may extract the virtues from the root. This may be used 3 or 4 times a day in doses of a table-spoon or more: and by adding a few drops of peppermint to this preparation, it is a good remedy to moderate puking which some-times occurs with pregnant women.

Serpentary is admirably suited to check vomiting and to tranquilize the stomach particularly in bilious cases. Steep the roots in warm water for a hour. Strain and drink in small doses as needed.

A tea made of black snake-root is very settling to the stomach, where persons are inclined to throw up their food.

In obstinate vomitings, helonias [infusion or decoction] frequently gives speedy relief, and that even in cases of pregnancy.

W. M. Hand, 1820

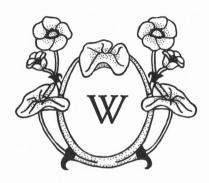

WARTS

Dissolve as much common washing soda as the water will take up, then wash the hands or warts with this for a minute or 2, and allow them to dry without being wiped. This repeated for 2 or 3 days, will gradually destroy the most irritable wart.

A solution of vinegar and baking soda will cure warts. If the wart is kept moist with it for 10 minutes 3 or 4 times a day, it will disappear in the course of a week or so.

Put on each wart, a small blister of Spanish flies, or lunar caustic, as in the case of corns: or you may wet the warts with a little sulphuric acid or oil of vitriol.

Rub wart with a slice of raw potato once or twice a day for a few days, and the wart will gradually disappear, without causing soreness, discoloring the skin, or leaving a scar.

Scrape a carrot fine, and mix with salt. Apply it as a poultice, for 5 or 6 nights.

Apply paste made of hickory ashes and strong vinegar.

The bark of the common willow burned to ashes and mixed with strong vinegar will remove warts or corns.

Oil of cinnamon dropped on warts 3 or 4 times a day will cause their disappearance, however hard, large, or dense they may be. The application gives no pain nor causes suppuration.

Warts may often be washed with a strong decoction of oak bark and will generally disappear under this treatment.

Rub the fresh cut Indian turnip root on wart several times daily.

Other applications: fresh juice of bloodroot, celandine, milkweed or fig tree.

WEIGHT

FOR THIN AND SCRAWNY CHILDREN

Give them from a teaspoon to a tablespoon pure olive oil after each meal. Give them a pinch of salt as soon as they have swallowed the olive oil, and no taste of the oil will remain in the mouth.

TO REDUCE WEIGHT OF ADULTS

A strong decoction of sassafras drink frequently, will reduce the flesh as rapidly as any remedy known. A strong infusion is made at the rate of an ounce of sassafras to a quart of water. Boil it ½ hour slowly, and let it stand till cold, heating again, if desired. Keep it from air.

Miss T. S. Shute, 1878

Take 1 ounce each of seawrack, sassafras, pipsissewa and wintergreen, ½ ounce of Epsom salts and the juice of 6 lemons. Steep the herbs for 1 hour, or until the strength is thoroughly extracted, strain and add the remaining ingredients. There should be 1 quart after it is fixed. Shake well before taking. The dose is a large tablespoonful the first thing before retiring. It is perfectly harmless and helps in more ways than the mere reduction of flesh. Taken as directed, as I say, it will surely do all that it is recommended to do; I judge from my own experience. The only food you must not eat is potato; with that single exception, you can eat what you want and as much as you care to. Don't sit down too much, and sleep and eat moderately; you will soon form the habit of doing things in this way, which is the proper one. The seawrack is probably the real flesh-reducing ingredient, but sassafras thins the blood and stimulates circulation, pipsissewa is excellent for kidneys, wintergreen serves as a flavoring, and we all know the virtues of lemon juice.

Century-old news item

The use of the leaves and stems of seawrack in decoction, powder, or pills will rapidly reduce the flesh, without discomfort or disturbance of the digestive functions.

J. King, M.D., 1864

Take 1 ounce seawrack, 1 ounce cleavers, ½ ounce motherwort. Mix, and place in 3 pints of water. Bring to a boil and simmer for 15 minutes. Strain when cold, and take ½ cupful after meals.

Drink a quart a day of a tea made with horehound herb.

Drink freely of an infusion made of chickweed herb.

A tea made of fennel seed was believed to lessen the sense of hunger.

The leaves of ash tree dried and prepared as a tea were used to reduce.

WEN

Wash in common salt water every day.

Wash with strong salt and vinegar twice a day for a month.

Take the yolks of eggs, beat up, and add as much fine salt as will dissolve, and apply a plaster to the wen every 10 hours. It cures without pain.

Paint with iodine (colorless tincture) daily or as often as it will bear application. This is slow but sure.

Apply oil of sassafras.

Take clean white linen rags, and burn them on some kind of pewter ware, and collect the oil of the rags on the pewter with lint. Cover the wen with this oil twice or 3 times a day. This must be continued for some time, and the wen will generally drop out without further trouble.

P. F. Bowker, 1836

WHOOPING COUGH

RECIPES USED TO ALLEVIATE THE
PAROXYSMS AND ALLEGED CURES

Take a big handful of oat straw, boil till it gets all the strength out; strain. Put in brown sugar, put back on the stove and make a syrup. Take it several times a day. It is good for a cough after one has whooping cough.

A teaspoonful of castor oil to a tablespoon of molasses; a teaspoon of the mixture to be given whenever the cough is troublesome. It will afford relief at once, and in a few days it effects a cure. The same remedy relieves the croup, however violent the attack.

Put hen's egg in a china cup and cover over with pure apple vinegar. Let it stand until the outer shell crumbles off like lime. Empty egg in vinegar and beat up and sweeten to taste with honey. Give as needed to loosen phlegm in small or large dose according to age of child. Repeat often.

Take 2 wineglasses of vinegar, 2 of honey, 2 of water, and 1 onion sliced. Simmer 1 hour. Dose 3 teaspoons night and morning for a child 8 years old.

Take ½ pound honey, 1 cup of water; let this boil, take off scum; pour boiling hot upon ½ ounce lobelia herb and ½ ounce of cloves; mix well, strain and add ¼ pint raspberry flavored vinegar. Take from 1 teaspoon to a dessertspoonful 4 times a day.

Take 1 gill each of garlic, sweet oil and honey, 1 ounce camphor; cook the garlic in the oil and strain and add the other ingredients. Take 1 teaspoon 3 or 4 times a day or as needed. This will cure the worst case.

Mrs. M. W. Ellsworth, 1897

A little saleratus, and occasionally a little bloodroot will be found greatly to alleviate the paroxysms.

Take 3 medium size leaves of prickly pear, cut up in pieces and place in a quart of cold water. Boil 30 minutes. Strain out all the prickles through close muslin or linen. Add sugar to the liquid, and boil a little longer. A safe and sure cure. Dose, from a teaspoon to tablespoon for a child as needed.

Boil 1 ounce mouse-ear herb in a pint of water for 3 minutes. Dose, a wineglass 3 or 4 times a day. Add a spoonful of brown sugar to each dose at the time of taking. This will work wonders. It is also a particularly good tonic for children.

The blooms of red clover steeped to a strong tea sweetened slightly is good for whooping cough. Give a swallow or 2 several times a day and give a dose of senna tea at bedtime.

Give an infusion made of pennyroyal herb sweetened with brown sugar.

Make a decoction of watermelon seed. Strain and add enough honey or brown sugar to make syrup.

The dried roots of marshmallow are very good being boiled in milk for the chin cough.

Yellow pond lily root, dried and pulverized, mixed with an equal quantity of honey, and taken a teaspoon at a time, several times in a day, will not only relieve the whooping cough, but will cure it in a short time.

Mrs. E. A. Howland, 1847

The skunk-cabbage root pulverized, is a valuable remedy in whooping cough. It is both loosening to the cough and quieting to the nerves, and may be given in doses of a ¼ or ½ teaspoon once or twice a day.

Unless there are complications, a tea or cough syrup made from chestnut leaves, and a laxative, are all that is necessary. Boil ½ ounce chestnut leaves to 1 pint of water. If syrup is preferred, add enough sugar to boil it down to proper consistency. Give as often as necessary. It is perfectly harmless, but needs a laxative occasionally.

Take elecampane root, 4 ounces; honey ½ a pound; set it in a warm place until it forms a syrup. Take 1 teaspoon 3 times a day.

Dr. A. A. Benezet, 1826

EXTERNAL APPLICATIONS

A sniff of turpentine will often ward off a bout of coughing or rub the chest with oil of eucalyptus.

Rub the feet thoroughly with hog's lard, before the fire, on going to bed, and keep the child warm therein. Or, rub the back, at lying down, with old rum: it seldom fails.

Take sweet oil and brandy, simmered with 1 onion sliced, and anoint the spine, chest, and soles of the feet, night and morning.

WORMS

Salt and water are good to turn worms.

Sweetened milk, with a little alum added to it, is good to turn worms.

Give a dose or 2 of flour of sulphur, mixed with molasses or honey: it brings off the worms without anything else.

Take tobacco leaves, pound them up with honey, and lay them on the belly of the child, or grown person, at the same time administering a dose of some good physic.

Dr. A. A. Benezet, 1826

To destroy worms in sickness or health. Take a tablespoon of molasses, and mix it with a teaspoon of the rust of tin. This is a safe remedy.

P. F. Bowker, 1836

Double tansy (fresh herb) worn upon the necks of children expels worms. And, indeed, the virtues of this herb are such that no family ought long to remain without it.

J. Monroe, 1824

The seed of lavender cotton being pounded into powder, and taken as worm-seed, kills worms, not only in children, but also in people of riper years. The herb itself has the same effect, but is not so powerful as the seed.

Birch bark gets rid of worms. Take ⅛ teaspoon of the pulverized bark, take 2nd dose in about 2 weeks if necessary. The powdered bark may be put into capsule and swallowed with a little water.

Mrs. D. F. G., 1964

Take blue flag root, 1 pound to 1 pint of gin; take 1 tablespoon 3 times a day, before eating.

Carolina pink stands high as a cure for worms. A knowledge of its properties as a vermifuge, was communicated to a number of the faculty in Carolina, by the Cherokee Indians. The root may be given in powder from ½ to 2 teaspoons, 2 or 3 times a day, after which give a brisk cathartic.

P. E. Sanborn, 1836

Purslaine dried carefully, and made into a tea, is the best thing for worms ever known. It is an easy and safe remedy for children or grown persons, and will harm no one.

P. F. Bowker, 1836

Take a quantity of white ash sprouts, and a handful of wild white poplar bark, boil it in a gallon of water, down to 1 quart, then put in ½ pint West-India molasses, ½ pint of brandy, and give a child from 1 to 3 years old, 1 tablespoon 3 times a day, before eating. Continue this 1 week, and it is a sure cure.

Dr. L. Sperry, 1843

One of the simplest and best remedies to be given to children, if they are troubled with worms, is poplar bark. It can be bought at any drug store, and a little paper, costing 5¢, will often prevent sickness, and possibly save a large doctor's bill. Take a little pinch of the bark, about as much as one would naturally take up on the point of a penknife, and give it before breakfast; it has a clean, bitter taste, and there is no difficulty in getting a child to take it if you explain what it is for.

Mrs. M. W. Ellsworth, 1897

There are many things helpful to children troubled with worms. Take the bark of witch hazel or spotted alder [the same bush], steep it in a pewter vessel, let it boil on a moderate heat, very strong; a child of a year old can take a tablespoon; if older, take more, according to the age. Let him take it 4 times a day, for several days. It is sure and safe.

Take 1 ounce of powdered snakehead herb, 1 drachm aloes, and 1 drachm of prickly ash bark; powder these, and to ½ a teaspoon of this powder add a teaspoon of boiling water, and a teaspoon of molasses, and take this as a dose, night or morning, more or less, as the symptoms require.

Take the spiky tops of wormwood, the blows of tansy and the bark from the root of sassafras, pound them fine, and sift through a fine sieve. Then take the bright scales of iron from a smith's forge, 2 or 3 ounces; pound and mix this with the above carefully, so that the iron may be properly mixed with the composition. A small teaspoon is a dose for a grown person, every night and morning, on an empty stomach, for 3 days. It must be mixed with molasses. Physic the fourth day with any convenient physic.

The leaves of sage powdered fine, and mixed with a little honey, a teaspoon for a dose.

An infusion made with sage, taken before breakfast or on going to bed, is excellent for children with round or pin worms.

Take 1 ounce of each of sage, ginger and senna leaves, steep in ½ pint of gin, take 1 tablespoon 3 times a day, before eating.

An infusion of the leaves and flowers of peach tree is given to children to purge the belly and destroy worms.

One teaspoon of the syrup of peach blossoms, taken in a glass of water distilled from the leaves, or in which the leaves and worm-seed have been decocted, is a most safe and certain medicine for the worms in children.

For pinworms, tapeworms, roundworms and hookworms, make a decoction of wormseed and take with a liquid diet. Follow with a cathartic. The oil of this plant is too poisonous for home use.

Wormseed is one of the best native remedies we have for expelling worms from the intestines. A teaspoon of the powdered herb and seed united with peppermint herb, pounded fine for a child 2 or 3 years old may be taken, night and morning before eating, for 2 or 3 days, then follow it with the common physical powders or any other brisk cathartic.

P. E. Sanborn, 1836

PINWORMS

Eat huckleberries (fresh or preserved) over a 3 day period.

Give an injection of an infusion of fresh garlic for 2 or 3 nights in succession. The infusion is made with a small bunch of garlic in a pint of water reduced to ⅛ pint.

Make an infusion of spearmint. Inject some in the bowel every night for 1 week. Some may be taken internally at the same time.

Boil ½ ounce quassia chips or calumbo in 1 pint of water for 3 or 4 minutes. Strain and when lukewarm inject the decoction in rectum once a day.

Take the tops and blows of Canada thistles, and boil them in spring water, until the strength is out. Strain off the liquor, and simmer it down, until it becomes quite thick, add the same quantity of molasses, you have a syrup; give for a dose, a wineglass, for an adult, and repeat every hour until it operates, which rarely fails of clearing the patient of those troublesome creatures.

P. F. Bowker, 1836

TAPEWORMS

Boil 1 ounce male fern root [*Dryopteris filix-mas*] in 1½ pints of water till reduced to 1 pint. Dose for adults: take no food before retiring, and in the morning take a wineglassful of the liquor.

Refrain from supper and breakfast on following morning, and at 8 o'clock take ⅓ part of 200 minced pumpkin seeds, the shells of which have been removed by hot water; at 9 take another ⅓, at 10 the remainder, and follow it at 11 with strong dose of castor oil. Most harmless of all tapeworm recipes.

WOUNDS

The best simple remedy for surface wounds, such as cuts, abrasion of the skin, etc., is wood charcoal. Take a large coal from the fire, pulverize it, apply it to the wound, and cover the whole with a rag. The charcoal absorbs the fluid secreted by the wound, and lays the foundation of the scab; it also prevents the rag from irritating the flesh.

For fresh wounds, take 3 different kinds of herbs, you need not be particular what kinds, chew them, and apply the spittle to the wound. This remedy is good for man or beast. It is simple and easy being always at hand.

The surgeons of our revolutionary army, and also those of general

Wayne's army, who defeated the Indians in August, 1794, experienced the most happy effects from the application of poultices of slippery elm bark, to gun shot wounds, which were soon brought to a good suppuration, and to a disposition to heal. It was applied as the first remedy. When tendency to mortification was evident, this bark bruised and boiled in water, produced the most surprising good effects. After repeated comparative experiments with other emollient applications, as milk and bread, and a linseed poultice, its superiority was firmly established.

Elias Smith, Physician, 1826

Tincture of arnica is used for the washing of wounds, for compresses, etc. Arnica blossoms are gathered at the end of June or the beginning of July, and put in brandy or spirit. In about 3 days, the tincture may be used.

Old suppurating wounds, if washed with a decoction of sage, will quickly heal.

Among the Indian nations, the leaves of Jamestown weed are made much use of, especially in cases of wounds, contusions or bruises, ulcerations, and the bites of reptiles.

J. C. Gunn, M.D., 1830

Take fresh green ground ivy and pound it up—good applied to a fresh wound.

For old wounds, boil 2 handfuls of ground ivy with rock alum, about the quantity of 2 walnuts, in 3 quarts of spring water, till it comes to 2. Wash the wound with it twice a day, for ½ hour, bathing or fomenting with flannel as hot as can be borne by the patient. The use of this has been attended with great success.

For open wound take adder's tongue roots crushed in olive oil and use as a dressing.

Many people apply the bruised leaves of plantain to slight wounds, inflamed sores, and swellings, with a favorable effect.

The roots of spikenard are bruised or chewed and used as poultices for all kinds of wounds and ulcers by the Indians.

The leaves of healall are useful as an external application to bruises, wounds, ulcers, etc., and both leaves and roots may be made into a salve with lard, or butter, and applied to sores and swellings.

During the Civil War, American surgeons used the juice of calendula flowers for wounds. The mashed leaves of the plant were also used as a poultice on wounds.

The herb of foxglove is frequently used to heal any fresh or green wounds, the leaves being bruised and bound on. And the juice of the leaves are also used for old sores, to cleanse, dry and heal them.

A poultice of fresh colt's foot leaves is a superior remedy for inflamed wounds.

The leaves of true love bruised, are very effectual to heal green wounds, and also filthy old sores and ulcers.

The leaves of primroses make the finest salve to heal wounds ever known.

The leaves of houseleek make the best salve known for wounds.

Catnip herb is excellent mixed with fresh [unsalted] butter and sugar for a green [fresh] wound.

BRUISES

The best treatment of sprains and bruises is the application of water, of such temperature as is most agreeable. The degree of temperature varies with the temperature of the weather and the vigor of the circulation. In a hot day use cool or cold water. If the circulation is low use warm water. The bruised or sprained parts may be immersed in a pail of water, and gently pressed or manipulated with the hand or soft cloth for 10 or 15 minutes, or even longer in severe cases, after which wrap up the parts in cloth wet in cold water, and keep quiet. This treatment keeps down the inflammation, and in 9 cases out of 10 proves a speedy cure.

Bruise beneath nails: Plunge the finger into water as hot as can be borne. By so doing, the nail is softened, and yields so as to accommodate itself to the blood poured out beneath it, and the agony is soon diminished. The finger may then be wrapped in a bread and water poultice.

Everything a Lady Should Know, about 1880

A bruise may be treated with either heat or cold. Apply flannels wrung out of boiling water or ice water, and continue applications for ½ hour. If this is done immediately, there will be no discoloration. Arnica or witch hazel may be added to the cold water with good effect. Poultices of bread and vinegar are also good.

Take 1 part blue clay and 2 parts vinegar, and make into a paste, and bind on at night with a wet towel. One application is generally sufficient.

In the first place bind on tobacco leaf moistened, keep it on 1 hour; then take it off and put on weak lye or bathe in the same 15 minutes, then put on fine salt, keep it on an hour, and it will take the soreness out and prevent taking cold; then put on a healing salve, or plaster, and it will effect a cure.

A poultice made with bran, and the bruised herb pellitory-of-the-wall, mixed with sweet oil; will remove pain from bruised parts and severe contusions.

Immediately apply molasses spread on brown paper. Or, apply a plaster of chopped parsley herb mixed with butter.

Wormwood steeped in vinegar gives almost immediate relief to bruises or sprains.

The fresh green leaves of tansy pounded, are good and will allay swelling.

To hasten healing and remove pain of bruises apply compresses wet with a strong decoction made with valerian roots.

TO PREVENT SKIN DISCOLORING AFTER BRUISES

Apply a cloth wrung in very hot water and renew frequently until the pain ceases.

Apply immediately, or as soon as possible, a little dry starch of arrowroot, moistened with cold water, or rub over with table butter.

Sweet oil with a little spirits of turpentine will usually prevent the unsightly black and blue spot.

The mashed herb of hyssop applied to a bruise speedily mitigates the pain and prevents discoloration.

Wormwood macerated in boiling water and repeatedly applied to a bruise, by way of cataplasm, will not only remove the pain, but also prevent the swelling and discoloration of the part.

CUTS

It is a wise plan to keep a cup of alum water always convenient, so that sudden cuts or bruises can be bound up in a cloth wet in it. If treated thus they will heal quickly.

There is nothing better for a cut than powdered resin. Get a few cents' worth, pound it until it is quite fine, put it in a cast-off spice box, with perforated top, then you can easily sift it on the cut. Put a soft cloth around the injured member, and wet it with water once in a while; it will prevent inflammation or soreness.

Wash with a weak solution of baking soda and while wet sprinkle full of black pepper.

Make a pad of cobwebs and apply to cut.

Apply the moist surface of the inside coating or skin of the shell of a raw egg; it will adhere of itself, leave no scar, and heal without pain.

C. Kinsley, 1876

The oil obtained from the yolks of eggs is credited with wonderful healing properties in cases of cuts, bruises and the like, by some of the Eastern nations. The eggs are first boiled hard, when the yolk is easily removed. Crushed and carefully stirred over a hot fire, the oil separates, when it is ready for use. The eggs of water fowls have the most oil, but that obtained from the eggs of the common guinea hen is considered best.

Miss T. S. Shute, 1878

Saturate bandage with tincture of myrrh and apply to affected parts.

Oil of eucalyptus is one of the best antiseptic and healing drugs. If applied to a fresh cut it will seldom get sore, and will heal without pus.

The leaves of geranium are an excellent application for cuts, where the skin is rubbed off, and other wounds of that kind. One or 2 leaves must be bruised and applied to the parts, and the wound will be cicatrized in a short time.

A poultice of the mashed leaves of live-forever is good for fresh cuts or wounds.

The roots of comfrey answer a fine purpose for cuts and wounds.

Marshmallow roots are very good made into a salve with honey and rosin, for all fresh cuts or wounds, healing them immediately.

The pounded fresh leaves of yerba mansa are good for cuts and wounds.

Take a quantity of the bark of sumac root and boil for 2 hours; strain and add fresh lard to the liquid. Then boil till the water is all out. Apply as a salve 3 times a day.

EXCESSIVE BLEEDING

Styptics are astringent substances applied to wounds or other bleeding surfaces, to stop the flow of blood. They are often very useful, but cannot be relied on when a large artery is wounded, though they ought to be resorted to when the means of taking up and tying the bleeding vessel are not at hand. The following are considered among the best articles of this class:

Dried beef, cut thin, dried, and pulverized; or it may be burnt to a coal, and pulverized.

Sassafras leaves chewed fine and applied, is said to be better than anything else.

Mandrake root is also highly recommended by some.

Burnt bone, pulverized, is, by many, considered a valuable styptic.

A strong tea of hickory bark, (that kind termed pignut) is highly recommended by Dr. Hough, and others.

H. Howard, 1857

Powdered rosin is the best thing to stop bleeding from cuts. After the powder is sprinkled on, wrap the wound with a soft cotton cloth. As soon as the wound begins to feel feverish, keep the cloth wet with cold water.

Apply paste made with flour and vinegar.

Equal parts of flour and salt bound on with cloth.

Take linen or other rags, burn to charcoal and put it in the wound, and no more blood will come.

Mix ashes of linen with sharp vinegar and apply.

Wood soot applied to a fresh cut or wound, will stop the blood, and abate the pain at the same time.

Mrs. E. A. Howland, 1847

Apply wet or powdered tea leaves.

Bind wound with tobacco.

Take ripe puffballs, break them warily, and save the powder. Strew this on the wound and bind it on. This will stop the bleeding of an amputated limb.

The leaves of allheal or woundwort being bruised and applied to a fresh wound, will stop the bleeding and cure the wound.

Alum-roots [*Heuchera americana*] were used by the Indians in the Alleghany Mountains, in powder, as an external remedy in sores, wounds, ulcers, and even cancers. Roots are powerfully astringent.

Peach leaves dried and powdered, are good to stop blood and heal wounds.

An application of matico-leaf stopped the bleeding on the tongue of a bleeder where everything else failed.

The leaves of yarrow have been used since remote times to stop bleeding of wounds.

Take the dried and pulverized leaves of common wild sunflower, sprinkle a small quantity into a wound, and the blood will cease to flow almost instantly, unless an artery is severed.

Bistort [*Polygonum bistorta*] is one of the most powerful astringents in nature. It is good for all bleeding, whether internally or externally.

Mrs. A. Matteson, 1894

The leaves and bark of common willow are used to staunch bleeding wounds.

An ointment made from woad leaves is good for severe bleeding in fresh wounds.

NAIL WOUNDS

If the wound is produced by a rusty nail, or a similar cause, so as to be jagged, it will soon become very inflamed, and in such a case, it is recommended to smoke such a wound with burning wool or woolen cloth. Twenty minutes in the smoke of wool will take the pain out of the worst wound, and if repeated once or twice will allay the worst cause of inflammation arising from a wound.

The Modern Home Cook Book
and Family Physician, about 1880

Take the skin of pork, well molded; place between bandages and apply to the wound. Will draw out infection. Pork rind is kept in cellar for time of need. It is claimed that this application will also bring boils to a head.

When a nail or pin has been run into the foot, instantly bind on a rind of salt pork, and keep quiet till the wound is well. The lockjaw is often caused by such wounds, if neglected.

Take a handful of peach tree leaves and put them in about a cup of boiling water and let them steep for a few minutes. Then make a stiff mash of the leaves and bind it on as hot as it can be borne. This will relieve the pain in 5 or 10 minutes.

Mrs. B. B., 1956

Bibliography

ALLEN. *Grandma Allen's Collection of Recipes.* About 1820.

ANSHUTZ, E. P. *New and Old Forgotten Remedies.* 1900.

BARNUM, H. L. *Family Receipts: or, Practical Guide for the Husbandman and Housewife.* 1831.

BEACH, W., M.D. *The American Practice of Medicine.* 3 vols. 1833.

——. *The Family Physician: or, The Reformed System of Medicine.* 1843.

BENEZET, DR. A. A. *Family Physician.* 1826.

BIGELOW, JACOB, M.D. *American Medical Botany, Being a Collection of the Native Medicinal Plants of the United States.* Vol. I, 1817, vol. II, 1818, vol. III, 1820.

BOWKER, PIERPONT E. *The Indian Vegetable Family Instructer.* 1836.

BRADBURY, ROBERT, M.D. *Encyclopaedia of Practical Information and Universal Formulary.* About 1882.

BRIANTE, DR. JOHN GOODALE. *The Old Root and Herb Doctor.* 1870.

CAPRON, GEORGE, M.D., and SLACK, DAVID B., M.D. *New England Popular Medicine.* 1848.

CARVER, J. *Travels Through the Interior Parts of North America in the Years 1766, 1767, and 1768, by J. Carver, Esq., Captain of a Company of Provincial Troops During the Late War with France.* 2nd. ed. 1779.

CLARKE, MRS. ANNA. *The Ideal Cookery Book.* 1889.

COE, GROVER, M.D. *Concentrated Organic Medicines, Being a Practical Exposition of the Therapeutic Properties and Clinical Employment of the Combined Proximate Medicinal Constituents of Indigenous and Foreign Plants.* 1858.

COOKE, MISS M. C. *Three Meals a Day.* 1889.

CORNELIUS, MRS. MARY H. *The Young Housekeeper's Friend.* 1871.

COXE, JOHN REDMAN, M.D. *The American Dispensatory.* 1818.

DARLINGTON, WILLIAM, M.D. *American Weeds and Useful Plants.* 1860.

DAVIS, DR. W. O. *The Indian Household Medicine Guide.* 1882.

DUFFEY, MRS. E. B. *What Women Should Know.* 1882.

ELLSWORTH, MRS. M. W. *Queen of the Household.* 1897.

FOWLER, C. H., and DE PUY, W. H. *Home and Health and Home Economics.* 1880.

GOOD, PETER P. *The Family Flora and Materia Medica Botanica.* 2 vols. 1854.

GRIFFITH, ROBERT EGLESFELD, M.D. *Medical Botany: or, Descriptions of the More Important Plants Used in Medicine, with Their History, Properties and Mode of Administration,* 1847.

GUNN, JOHN C., M.D. *Gunn's Domestic Medicine: or, Poor Man's Friend.* Printed under the immediate superintendance of the author, a physician of Knoxville. 1st ed. 1830.

———. *Gunn's New Domestic Physician: or, Home Book of Health.* 1862.

HAND, WILLIAM M. *The House Surgeon and Physician: Designed to assist heads of families, travellers, and sea-faring people, in discerning, distinguishing, and curing diseases; with concise directions for the preparation and use of a numerous collection of the best American remedies; together with many of the most approved from the shop of the apothecary. All in plain English.* 2nd ed., revised and enlarged. 1820.

HOLLENBACK, H. *American Eclectic Materia Medica.* 1865.

HOWARD, HORTON. *An Improved System of Domestic Medicine.* 1857.

HOWLAND, MRS. E. A. *The New England Economical Housekeeper and Family Receipt Book.* 1847.

JAMES, DR. B. W. *Note Book of Recipes.* 1852.

KALM, PETER, *Travels into North America.* 2 vols. 1772.

KING, JOHN, M.D. *The American Eclectic Dispensatory.* 1855.

———. *The American Family Physician: or, Domestic Guide to Health.* 1864.

KINSLEY, CHARLES. *The Circle of Useful Knowledge, For the Use of Farmers, Mechanics, Merchants, Manufacturers, Surveyors, Housekeepers, Professional Men, Etc.* 1876.

LOUIS, DR. R. L. *Our Home Counselor.* 1877.

MARQUART, JOHN. *Six Hundred Receipts.* 1867.

MATTESON, MRS. ANTONETTE. *The Occult Family Physician and Botanic Guide to Health.* 1894.

MATTSON, M., M.D. *The American Vegetable Practice: or, A New and Improved Guide to Health, Designed for the Use of Families.* 1841.

MILLSPAUGH, CHARLES F., M.D. *American Medical Plants.* 3 vols. 1887.

MONROE, JOHN. *The American Botanist and Family Physician.* 1824.

NEILL, MISS E. *Complete Encyclopedia of Cookery and Practical Recipes.* 1890.

OWENS. *Mrs. Owens' New Cook Book.* 1897.

PANCOAST, S., M.D. *The Ladies' New Medical Guide.* 1901.

PEREIRA, JONATHAN, M.D., F.R.S. and L.S. *The Elements of Materia Medica and Therapeutics.* 2 vols. 1846.

PORTER, MRS. M. E. *New World Fair Cook Book.* 1891.

RAFINESQUE, C. S., A.M. PH.D. *Medical Flora: or, Manual of the Medical Botany of the United States of North America.* Vol. I, 1828, vol. II, 1830.

ROGERS, DR. DAVID. *The American Physician, Being a New System of Practice Founded on Botany.* 1824.

SANBORN, P. E. *The Sick Man's Friend, Being a Plain, Practical Medical Work, Designed for the Use of Families and Individuals on Vegetable or Botanical Principles.* 1836.

SCUDDER, JOHN M., M.D. *Specific Medication and Specific Medicines.* 1873.

SHUTE, MISS T. S. *The American Housewife Cook Book.* 1878.

SMITH, DR. DANIEL. *The Reformed Botanic Indian Physician.* 1855.

SMITH, ELIAS, PHYSICIAN. *The American Physician and Family Assistant.* 1826.

SMITH, ELISHA, PHYSICIAN AND SURGEON. *The Botanic Physician.* 1830.

SMITH, PETER. *The Indian Doctor's Dispensatory, Being Father Smith's Advice respecting Diseases and Their Cure.* 1812.

SPERRY, D. L. *The Botanic Family Physician: or, The Secret of Curing Diseases.* 1843.

STOUT, H. R., M.D. *Our Family Physician.* 1886.

THOMSON, SAMUEL. *A Narrative of the Life and Medical Discoveries of Samuel Thomson, Containing an Account of His System of Practice.* 1829.

——. *New Guide to Health: or, Botanic Physician.* 1831.

WOOD, GEORGE P., M.D., and RUDDOCK, E. H., M.D. *Vitalogy: or, Encyclopedia of Health and Home.* 1899.

UNKNOWN AUTHORS

Everything a Lady Should Know. About 1880.

Practical Housekeeping. The Buckeye Publishing Company, 1887.

The Buckeye Cook Book. The Buckeye Publishing Company, 1876.

The Housewife's Library. 1885.

The Kansas Home Cook Book. 1879.

The Modern Home Cook Book and Family Physician. About 1880.

The Gem Cook Book, by a New England Lady. 1875.

Common and Latin Names
of Plants

Adam's flannel *Verbascum thaspus*
Adder's tongue *Erythronium americanum*
Agrimony *Agrimonia eupatoria*
Ague weed *Eupatorium perfoliatum*
Allheal *Prunella vulgaris*
Aloe barbadensis *Aloe vulgaris* or *A. vera*
Alum root *Geranium maculatum*
Alum-root *Heuchera americana*
American brooklime *Veronica americana*
American valerian *Cypripedium luteum* or *C. pubescens*
Angelica, American *Angelica sylvestris*
Angelica, European *Angelica archangelica*
Aniseed *Pimpinella anisum*
Anise-scented goldenrod *Solidago odora*
Arnica *Arnica montana*
Arrowroot *Maranta arundinacea*
Arsmart *Polygonum punctatum*
Asafoetida *Ferula foetida*
Ash, black or yellow *Fraxinus nigra*
Ash, white *Fraxinus alba, F. acuminata* or *F. americana*
Asthma weed *Lobelia inflata*
August flower *Amphiachyris dracunculoides*
Avens *Geum rivale*

Balm *Melissa officinalis*
Balm of gilead *Populus balsamifera*

Balmony   *Chelone glabra*
Balsam fir or pitch   *Abies nigra*
Barberry   *Berberis vulgaris*
Basswood   *Tilia americana*
Bayberry   *Myrica cerifera*
Bearberry   *Arctostaphylos uva-ursi*
Beech drops   *Orobanche virginianum*
Beech tree   *Fagus grandifolia*
Benne or bene   *Sesamum indicum*
Beth-root   *Trillium cernum, T. erectum* or *T. pendulum*
Betony, European   *Betonica officinalis*
Birch, black   *Betula nigra*
Birch, red   *Betula lenta*
Birch, white   *Betula alba*
Birthroot   *Trillium erectum*
Bistort   *Polygonum bistorta*
Biting arsmart   *Polygonum punctata*
Bitter root or American gentian   *Gentiana catesbaei*
Bitterroot or Indian hemp   *Apocynum androsaemifolium*
    or *A. cannabinum*
Bittersweet bark of root   *Celastrus scandens*
Bittersweet twigs   *Solanum dulcamara*
Bitter thistle   *Cnicus benedictus*
Black alder   *Ilex verticillata*
Blackberry   *Rubus fruticosus*
Blackberry brier   *Rubus canadensis*
Black cohosh or cohush   *Cimicifuga racemosa*
Black elder   *Sambucus canadensis*
Black haw   *Viburnum prunifolium*
Black horehound   *Ballota foetida*
Black larch   *Larix laricina*
Black maple   *Acer nigrum*
Black pussywillow   *Salix nigra*
Black raspberry   *Rubus occidentalis*
Black root   *Leptandra virginica*
Black snakeroot   *Sanicula marilandica*
Black spruce   *Abies nigra*
Black walnut   *Juglans nigra*
Black willow   *Salix nigra*
Bladderwrack   *Fucus vesiculosus*
Blessed thistle   *Cnicus benedictus*
Bloodroot   *Sanguinaria canadensis*
Blood weed   *Erigeron canadensis*
Blueberry   *Caulophyllum thalictroides*
Blue cohosh or cohush   *Caulophyllum thalictroides*

Blue flag   *Iris versicolor*
Blue vervain   *Verbena hastata*
Boldo   *Peumus boldus*
Boneset   *Eupatorium perfoliatum*
Brierroot   *Smilax pseudo-china*
Broomcorn   *Sorghum saccharatum*
Broom tops or herb   *Cytisus scoparius*
Buchu   *Barosma crenulata*
Buckbean   *Menyanthes trifoliata*
Buckeye   *Aesculus glabra*
Buckhorn brake   *Osmunda regalis*
Buckthorn, American   *Rhamnus caroliniana*
Buckthorn, European   *Rhamnus cathartica*
Bugle weed   *Lycopus virginicus*
Bull nettle   *Solanum carolinense*
Bull thistle   *Carduus lanceolatus*
Burdock   *Arctium lappa*
Butternut   *Juglans cinerea*
Button snakeroot   *Eryngium aquaticum*
Button weed   *Diodella rigida*

Cajuput, cajaput, or cajeput   *Melaleuca leucadendron*
Calamus   *Acorus calamus*
Calendula   *Calendula officinalis*
Canada fleabane   *Erigeron canadensis*
Canada thistle   *Cirsium arvense*
Cancer root   *Orobanche virginianum*
Cancer weed   *Salvia lyrata*
Canella   *Canella alba*
Cape aloes   *Aloe ferox*
Caraway seed   *Carum carvi*
Cardamon seed   *Elettaria cardamomum*
Carolina pink   *Spigelia marilandica*
Carpenter square   *Scrophularia marilandica*
Cascara (sagrada)   *Rhamnus purshiana*
Catechu   *Acacia catechu*
Catnip   *Nepeta cataria*
Cat-tail or cat-tail flag   *Typha latifolia*
Cayenne or chili pepper   *Capsicum frutescens*
Celandine or celendyne   *Chelidonium majus*
Centaury   *Erythraea Centaurium*
Chamomile or camomile   *Matricaria chamomilla*
Checkerberry   *Gaultheria procumbens*
Cheese plant   *Malva rotundifolia*

Chestnut   *Castanea dentata*
Chickweed   *Stellaria media*
Chicory   *Cichorium intybus*
China root   *Rheum officinale*
Cicuta   *Cicuta maculata*
Cinchona   *Cinchona officinalis*
Cinquefoil   *Potentilla canadensis*
Clary   *Salvia sclarea*
Cleareye   *Salvia sclarea*
Cleavers or clivers   *Galium aparine*
Cocash   *Aster puniceus*
Cockleburs   *Xanthium spinosum*
Cold water root   *Aster puneceus*
Colic root   *Dioscorea villosa*
Coltsfoot   *Tussilago farfara*
Colombo, columbo, or calumbo, American   *Frasera carolinensis*
Comfrey   *Symphytum officinale*
Coneflower   *Echinacea angustifolia*
Coral bean   *Erythrina herbacea*
Coriander seed   *Coriandrum sativum*
Corn silk   *Zea mays*
Cotton plant   *Gossypium herbaceum*
Couch grass   *Agropyron repens*
Coughwort   *Tussilago farfara*
Cow parsnip   *Heracleum lanatum*
Cowslip   *Primula veris*
Crab apple   *Pyrus coronaria*
Cramp bark   *Viburnum opulus*
Cranberry   *Vaccinium macrocarpon*
Crane's-bill or cranesbill   *Geranium maculatum*
Creosote bush   *Larrea divaricata*
Crow corn   *Aletris farinosa*
Cubebs   *Piper cubeba*
Cudweed   *Gnaphalium uliginosum*
Culver's root   *Leptandra virginica*
Cumin   *Cuminum cyminum*
Currant   *Ribes floridum*
Currant, black   *Ribes nigrum*
Currant, red   *Ribes rubrum*

Dandelion   *Taraxacum officinale*
Deer's tongue   *Erythonium americanum*
Devil's bit   *Leatris spicata*

Dewberry   *Rubus canadensis*
Dill seed   *Anethum gravolens*
Dittany or ditany   *Cunila origanoides*
Dogbane   *Apocynum androsaemifolium*
Dog-fennel   *Eupatorium capillifolium*
Dog grass   *Agropyron repens*
Dog mackimus   *Cornus circinata*
Dogwood   *Cornus florida*
Dollar vine   *Rhynchosia tomentosa*
Dragon root   *Arisaema dracontium*
Dwarf elder   *Sambucus ebulus*

Echinacea   *Echinacea angustifolia*
Elder, common   *Sambucus canadensis*
Elecampane   *Inula helenium*
Emetic herb   *Lobelia inflata*
Emetic root   *Euphorbia corollata*
English saffron   *Carthamus tinctorius*
Erigeron   *Erigeron canadensis*
Eucalyptus   *Eucalyptus globulus*
Eyebright   *Euphrasia officinalis*

False bittersweet   *Celastrus scandens*
False saffron   *Carthamus tinctorius*
Female flowers   *Senecio aureus*
Female regulator   *Senecio aureus*
Fennel   *Foeniculum vulgare*
Fenugreek   *Trigonella foenum-graecum*
Fever-bush   *Benzoin aestivale*
Feverfew   *Chrysanthemum parthenium*
Field thistle   *Cirsium arvense*
Fig   *Ficus carica*
Figwort   *Scrophularia marilandica*
Fir balsam   *Abies nigra*
Fireweed   *Erechtites hieracifolia*
Five-finger-grass   *Potentilla canadensis*
Flaxseed   *Linum usitatissimum*
Fleabane   *Erigeron canadensis*
Flowering dogwood   *Cornus florida*
Foxglove   *Digitalis purpurea*
Fringe tree   *Chionanthus virginica*
Fumitory   *Fumaria officinalis*

Galangal   *Alpinia officinarum*
Garget   *Phytolacca decandra*
Gentian   *Gentiana lutea*
Geranium root   *Geranium maculatum*
Germander   *Teucrium chamaedrys*
Ginseng   *Panax quinquefolia*
Globe flower   *Cephalantus occidentalis*
Gobernadora   *Larrea divaricata*
Goldenrod   *Solidago rigida* or *S. virgaurea*
Golden seal   *Hydrastis canadensis*
Gold-thread   *Coptis trifolia*
Gooseberry   *Ribes uva-crispa*
Grape vine   *Vitis vinifera*
Gravel weed   *Epigaea repens*
Green ozier   *Cornus circinata*
Ground hemlock   *Taxus minor*
Ground ivy   *Glechoma hederacea*
Ground pine   *Lycopodium clavatum*
Guaiac   *Guaiacum officinalis*
Guarana   *Paullina cupana*
Gum plant   *Grindelia robusta* or *G. squarrosa*

Hair-cap moss   *Polytrichum junipernum*
Hawthorn berries   *Crataegus oxyacantha*
Healall   *Scrophularia marilandica*
Heart's ease or pansy   *Viola tricolor*
Hedge mustard   *Sisymbrium officinale*
Hellebore   *Veratrum viride*
Helonias   *Chamaelirium luteum*
Hemlock tree   *Tsuga canadensis*
Hens-and-chickens   *Sempervivum tectorum*
Hickory   *Carya alba*
High mallow   *Althaea officinalis*
Hollyhock   *Althaea rosea*
Holy thistle   *Cnicus benedictus*
Honeysuckle   *Diervilla canadensis*
Hops   *Humulus lupulus*
Horehound   *Marrubium vulgare*
Horse-balm   *Collinsonia canadensis*
Horse chestnut   *Aesculus hippocastanum*
Horsemint   *Monarda punctata*
Horseradish   *Cochlearia armoracia*
Horsetail   *Equisetum hyemale* or *E. arvense*

Houseleek   *Sempervivum tectorum*
Hyssop   *Hyssopus officinalis*

Iceland moss   *Cetraria islandica*
Indian cup-plant   *Silphium perfoliatum*
Indian hemp   *Apocynum androsaemifolium* or *A. cannabinum*
Indigo or indigofera   *Baptisia tinctoria* or *B. alba*
Ipecac   *Cephaelis ipecacuanha*
Ipecac, wild   *Euphorbia corollata*
Irish moss   *Chondrus crispus*

Jack-in-the-pulpit   *Arisaema triphyllum*
Jacob's ladder   *Polemonium reptans*
Jalap   *Impomoea purga*
Jalap, wild   *Impomoea hederacea* or *I. pandurata*
Jamaica ginger   *Zingiber officinale*
Jamaica sarsaparilla   *Smilax regelii*
Jamestown or jimson weed   *Datura stramonium*
Jerusalem oak   *Chenopodium botrys*
Jewelweed   *Impatiens biflora* or *I. pallida*
Jill-grow-over-the-ground   *Glechoma hederacea*
Job's tears   *Coix lacryma-jobi*
Joe-pye weed or joepye   *Eupatorium purpureum*
Juniper berries   *Juniperus communis*

Kava kava   *Piper methysticum*
Kelp   *Macrocystis pyrifera*
Kidney liver-leaf   *Hepatica americana*
Kidney root   *Eupatorium purpureum*
Kidneywort   *Hepatica acutiloba*
Knotgrass   *Polygonum aviculare*

Lady's slipper   *Cypripedium luteum* or *C. pubescens*
Larch, European   *Larix decidua*
Laurel   *Magnolia virginiana* or *M. glauca*
Lavender   *Lavandula officinalis*
Lavender cotton   *Santolina chamaecyparissus*
Leatherbush   *Dirca palustris*
Lemon balm   *Melissa officinalis*
Licorice   *Glycyrrhiza glabra*

Life everlasting   *Gnaphalium polycephalum*
Life-of-man root   *Aralia racemosa*
Life root   *Senecio aureus*
Lily-of-the-valley   *Convallaria majalis*
Lime flowers   *Tilia europaea*
Linden, European   *Tilia europaea*
Linwood   *Tilia americana*
Live-forever or livelong   *Sedum telephium*
Liverwort   *Hepatica acutiloba* or *H. triloba*
Logwood   *Haematoxylon campechianum*
Lovage   *Levisticum officinale*
Low balm   *Monarda didyma*
Low mallow   *Malva rotundifolia*

Maidenhair fern   *Adiantum pedatum*
Mallow   *Malva sylvestris*
Mallows   *Malva rotundifolia*
Manchineel   *Hippomane mancinella*
Mandrake, American   *Podophyllum peltatum*
Manna   *Fraxinus ornus*
Man-root   *Ipomoea pandurata*
Maple   *Acer* species
Marigold   *Calendula officinalis*
Marjoram   *Origanum vulgare*
Marshmallow   *Althaea officinalis*
Marsh rosemary   *Limonium carolinianum*
Masterwort   *Imperatoria ostruthium*
Matico-leaf   *Piper angustifolium*
Mayapple   *Podophyllum peltatum*
Mayweed   *Maruta cotula*
Meadow-sweet, American   *Spiraea tomentosa*
Meadow-sweet, European   *Spiraea ulmaria*
Milkweed root   *Asclepias syriaca*
Mistletoe   *Viscum album*
Moosewood   *Acer nigrum*
Motherwort   *Leonurus cardiaca*
Mountain ash   *Sorbus aucuparia*
Mountain cranberry   *Arctostaphylos uva-ursi*
Mountain dittany   *Cunila origanoides*
Mountain grape   *Mahonia aquifolium*
Mountain mint   *Koellia virginiana*
Mouse-ear   *Gnaphalium uliginosum*
Mugwort   *Artemisia vulgaris*
Mulberry, black   *Morus nigra*

Mulberry, red   *Morus rubra*
Mulberry, white   *Morus alba*
Mullein or mullen   *Verbascum thapsus*
Musk root   *Malva moschata*
Myrrh   *Balsamodendron myrrha*

Nephritic plant   *Parthenium integrifolium*
Nettles   *Urtica dioica*
Nightshade   *Solanum nigrum*
Nine bark   *Physocarpus opulifolius*
Nosebleed   *Achillea millefolium*

Oats   *Avena sativa*
Oregon grape   *Mahonia aquifolium*

Palmetto berries   *Serenoa serrulata*
Paprika   *Capsicum annum*
Pareira brava   *Cissampelos pareira*
Parsley, garden   *Apium petroselinum*
Parsley piert   *Alchemilla arvensis*
Peach   *Prunus persica*
Pellitory-of-the-wall   *Parietaria officinalis*
Pennyroyal   *Hedeoma pulegioides*
Peony   *Paeonia officinalis*
Peppermint   *Mentha piperita*
Peruvian bark   *Cinchona officinalis*
Pig-nut hickory   *Carya parcena* or *C. glabra*
Pigweed   *Chenopodium album*
Pilewort   *Scrophularia marilandica*
Pipsissewa or pipsisway   *Chimaphila umbellata*
Pitch pine   *Pinus palustris*
Plantain   *Plantago major*
Pleurisy root   *Asclepias tuberosa*
Poison hemlock   *Cicuta maculata*
Poke   *Phytolacca decandra*
Polypody brake   *Polypodium vulgare*
Poplar   *Populus tremuloides*
Poppy, wild   *Argemone mexicana* or *A. alba*
Prickly ash   *Xanthoxylum americanum*
Prickly pear   *Opuntia vulgaris*
Primrose   *Primula vulgaris*
Primula   *Primula veris*

Prince's feather *Amaranthus hypochondriacus*
Prince's pine or prince of pine *Chimaphila umbellata*
Privet bush *Ligustrum vulgare*
Puffballs *Calvatia* species
Puke-weed *Lobelia inflata*
Pulsatilla *Anemone pulsatilla*
Purple loosestrife *Lythrum salicaria*
Purslane or purslaine *Portulaca oleracea*
Pussy willow *Salix nigra*
Pyrola *Pyrola americana*
Pyrole *Chimaphila umbellata*

Quaking aspen *Populus tremuloides*
Quassia chips *Quassia amara*
Queen-of-the-meadow root *Eupatorium purpureum*
Queen of the meadow tops *Spiraea salicifolia*
Quince *Cydonia oblonga*

Rabbit-tobacco *Gnaphalium polycephalum*
Ragweed *Ambrosia artemisiifolia*
Ragwort *Senecio aureus*
Rattleroot *Cimicifuga racemosa*
Rattlesnake plantain *Goodyera pubescens*
Rattlesnake's master *Eryngium aquaticum*
Red alder *Alnus rubra*
Red bark *Cinchona officinalis*
Red birthroot *Trillium erectum*
Red cedar *Juniperus virginiana*
Red centuary *Sabatia angularis*
Red clover *Trifolium pratense*
Red oak *Quercus rubra*
Red puccon root *Sanguinaria canadensis*
Red raspberry *Rubus idaeus*
Red root *Ceanothus americana*
Red willow *Cornus amomum*
Rhatany *Krameria triandra*
Rheumatism-weed *Chimaphila umbellata*
Rhubarb *Rheum officinale*
Ribwort *Plantego lanceolata*
Rocky mountain grape *Mahonia aquifolium*
Rosemary *Rosmarinus officinalis*
Rose petals *Rosa damascena* or *R. gallica*
Rose willow *Cornus amomium*

Rue   *Ruta graveolens*
Rupturewort   *Herniaria glabra*

Sacred bark   *Rhamnus purshiana*
Saffron, false   *Carthamus tinctorius*
Saffron, true   *Crocus sativus*
St. John's bread   *Ceratonia siliqua*
St. John's wort   *Hypericum perforatum*
Samphire   *Salicornia ambigua*
Sandalwood   *Santalum album*
Sanicle   *Sanicula marilandica*
Sarsaparilla   *Smilax officinalis*
Sarsaparilla, American   *Aralia nudicaulis*
Sassafras   *Sassafras albidum* or *S. variifolium*
Savin   *Juniperus virginiana*
Saw palmetto   *Serenoa serrulata*
Scarlet sumach   *Rhus glabra*
Scoke or poke   *Phytolacca decandra*
Scurry-grass   *Cochlearia officinalis*
Sea onion   *Urginea maritima*
Seawrack or bladderwrack   *Fucus vesiculosus*
Sedge grass   *Cyperus ovularis*
Selfheal   *Prunella vulgaris*
Seneca or senega snakeroot   *Polygala senega*
Senna, American   *Cassia marilandica*
Senna, Egyptian   *Cassia angustifolia*
Serpentary   *Aristolochia serpentaria*
Sesame   *Sesamum indicum*
Shavegrass   *Equisetum arvense*
Sheepberry   *Viburnum lentago*
Sheep's sorrel   *Rumex acetosella*
Shepherd's purse   *Capsella bursa-pastoris*
Silver grass   *Chrysopsis gramminifolia*
Silverweed   *Potentilla anserina*
Skullcap or scullcap   *Scutellaria lateriflora*
Skunk cabbage   *Symplocarpus foetidus*
Slippery elm   *Ulmus fulva*
Smallage   *Apium graveolens*
Smartweed   *Polygonum punctatum* or *P. hydropiper*
Smellage   *Levisticum officinale*
Snakehead or snake's head   *Chelone glabra*
Snakeroot   *Aristolochia serpentaria*
Snakeroot, Canada   *Asarum canadense*
Sneezeweed   *Helenium autumnale*

Soapwort   *Saponaria officinalis*
Socotrine aloes   *Aloe perryi*
Solomon's seal   *Convallaria multiflora*
Sorrel plant   *Rumex acetosella*
Sorrel tree   *Andromeda arborea*
Southernwood   *Artemisia abrotanum*
Sow thistle   *Sonchus oleraceus*
Spearmint   *Mentha viridis*
Speedwell   *Veronica officinalis*
Spicebush or spicewood   *Benzoin aestivale*
Spikenard or spignard   *Aralia racemosa*
Spleenwort   *Asplenium trichomanes*
Spruce   *Abies nigra*
Squaw root   *Cimicifuga racemosa*
Squaw vine   *Mitchella repens*
Squaw weed   *Senecio aureus*
Squills   *Urginea maritima*
Star root   *Aletris farinosa*
Stillingia   *Stillingia sylvatica*
Stinging nettle   *Urtica dioica*
Stone root   *Collinsonia canadensis*
Strawberry   *Fragaria virginiana*
Sumac or sumach   *Rhus glabra*
Sunflower   *Helianthus annuus*
Swamp sumac or poison sumac   *Rhus vernix*
Sweet balm   *Melissa officinalis*
Sweet elder   *Sambucus canadensis*
Sweet fern   *Comptonia asplenifolia*
Sweet flag   *Acorus calamus*
Sweet gum   *Liquidambar styraciflua*
Sycamore   *Plantanus occidentalis*
Syria grass   *Sorghum* species

Tag alder   *Alnus serrulata*
Tamarack or tamarac   *Larix americana*
Tansy   *Tanacetum vulgare*
Thimble-berry   *Rubus occidentalis*
Thimble-weed   *Anemone virginiana*
Thoroughwort   *Eupatorium perfoliatum*
Throatroot   *Geum rivale*
Thuja   *Thuja occidentalis*
Thyme   *Thymus vulgaris*
Toadflax   *Linaria vulgaris*
Toothache-tree   *Xanthoxylum americanum*

Tormentil *Potentilla tormentilla*
Trailing arbutus *Epigaea repens*
True love *Trillium erectum*
Tulip tree *Liriodendron tulipifera*
Turkey root or Turkey rhubarb *Rheum officinale*
Twinleaf *Jeffersonia diphylla*

Umbil root *Cypripedium parviflorum*
Unicorn *Aletris farinosa*
Uva-ursi *Arctostaphylos uva-ursi*

Valerian *Valeriana officinalis*
Vervain *Verbena hastata*
Viburnum *Viburnum prunifolium*
Violet, birdfoot or crowfoot *Viola pedata*
Violet, blue *Viola cucullata*
Violet, common *Viola rotundifolia*
Viper's bugloss *Echium vulgare*
Virginia snakeroot *Aristolochia serpentaria*

Wahoo *Euonymus atropurpureus* or *E. americanus*
Walnut, black *Juglans nigra*
Walnut, white *Juglans cinerea*
Water avens *Geum rivale*
Water cress *Radicula officinalis*
Water dock *Rumex aquaticus*
White alder *Clethra alnifolia*
White bean *Phaseolus vulgaris*
White beech *Fagus grandiflora*
White birthroot *Trillium cernuum* or *T. grandiflorum*
White cohosh or cohush *Actaea alba*
White hellebore *Veratrum viride*
White melilot *Melilotus alba*
White oak *Quercus alba*
White pine *Pinus strobus*
White plantain *Plantago virginica*
White pond lily *Castalia odorata*
White poplar, bark of root *Liriodendron tulipifera*
White poplar, bark of tree trunk *Populus tremuloides*
White root *Asclepias tuberosa*
White swamp honeysuckle *Rhododendron viscosum*
White wood, bark of root *Liriodendron tulipifera*

Whitlow grass   *Draba verna*
Whortleberry or whortle bush   *Vaccinium arboreum*
Wicky   *Sorbus aucuparia*
Wild angelica   *Angelica sylvestris*
Wild carrot   *Daucus carota*
Wild celandine   *Impatiens pallida*
Wild chamomile   *Maruta cotula*
Wild cherry   *Prunus serotina*
Wild ginger   *Asarum canadense*
Wild ipecac   *Euphorbia corollata*
Wild jalap   *Ipomoea hederacea* or *I. pandurata*
Wild leek   *Allium tricoccum*
Wild lettuce   *Lactuca canadensis*
Wild licorice   *Aralia nudicaulis*
Wild marjoram   *Origanum vulgare*
Wild mint   *Mentha canadensis*
Wild onion   *Allium stellatum*
Wild plum   *Prunus spinosa*
Wild sage   *Salvia lyrata*
Wild succory   *Cichorium intybus*
Wild white daisy   *Chrysanthemum leucanthemum*
Wild yam   *Dioscorea villosa*
Willow, common   *Salix alba* or *S. nigra*
Windflower   *Anemone virginiana*
Wintergreen   *Gaultheria procumbens*
Witch hazel   *Hamamelis virginiana*
Woad   *Isatis tinctoria*
Wood betony   *Pedicularis canadensis*
Wood sage   *Teucrium canadense*
Wood sorrel   *Oxalis acetosella*
Wormseed   *Chenopodium anthelminticum*
Wormwood   *Artemisia absinthium*
Woundwort   *Prunella vulgaris*

Yarrow   *Achillea millefolium*
Yellow dock   *Rumex crispus*
Yellow melilot   *Melilotus officinalis*
Yellow oak   *Quercus castanea*
Yellow parilla   *Menispermum canadense*
Yellow pond lily   *Nelumbo lutea*
Yellow root   *Xanthoriza apiifolia*
Yerba de pasmo   *Baccharis pteronioides*
Yerba mansa   *Anemopsis californica*